Living with
Huntington's
Disease

Living with Huntington's Disease

A Book for Patients and Families

Dennis H. Phillips

with a foreword by
Marjorie Guthrie

The University of Wisconsin Press

Published 1982

The University of Wisconsin Press
114 North Murray Street
Madison, Wisconsin 53715

The University of Wisconsin Press, Ltd.
1 Gower Street
London WC1E 6HA, England

First printing

Printed in the United States of America

For LC CIP information see the colophon

ISBN 0-299-08670-4 cloth, 0-299-08674-7 paperback

FOR WOODY, MARJORIE, AND JEBBY

*It is better to light one candle
than to curse the darkness.*

Contents

Figures

Foreword

In 1967, I sat reading in the National Airport in Washington, D.C., with tears streaming down my face. I had come to the National Institutes of Health, looking for someone to tell me something about Huntington's chorea. I had met Dr. Richard Masland, the Director of the Neurology Institute, who told me that we know very little about this rare disease. He then sent me to meet Dr. Ntinos Myrianthopoulos, who had just published his monograph on Huntington's the year before. I was devastated as I read each section. My husband Woody lay dying in a mental hospital, his illness diagnosed as Huntington's chorea. My three little children were at home. I had no one to talk to, and when I finally boarded the plane to return to New York City I felt weak and the words "hopeless and helpless" were ringing in my ears. Reading the hereditary aspects troubled me the most. How could I live knowing that any or all of my children might inherit their father's disease?

Woody had been hospitalized almost fifteen years. But as I had watched the slow progressive onslaught of his disease, I had learned some things about Huntington's, I thought, that some of the doctors who had painted such a bleak picture didn't know. I observed that Woody did not become the "vegetable" that I expected to see, and that although he could no longer walk or talk, he seemed quite responsive as he managed to answer my questions through a card system that we had developed. He was obviously happy to see me when I came to visit, and I wondered if the doctor realized how intact he really was!

Today, as I finished reading Dennis Phillips's manuscript, all I could think of was, if only *this* book had been given to me on that terrifying day just about fourteen years ago! Reading each section, learning about what Huntington's is and what it is not and how people are meeting the challenge of HD, could have spared me so much sadness. Dennis has included the thinking of many people, because Huntington's has become a topic of great interest in the medical and scientific community. It is good to explore genetic counseling and to allow those of us who are interested to know what the social problems are and how the health professionals are working together with the HD families and organizations to help our loved ones to live with HD through each stage of the progression.

Here is information about the kind of research that is going on in laboratories around the world. There is a section on the experimental treatments, and while there are no answers to what causes HD or why the gene begins to express itself at some time in each person's life, there is a wonderful feeling of hope. Hope because dedicated people *do* care. The network of scientific researchers, health professionals, friends, and HD families are all joining forces with governmental agencies and are saying, "You are no longer alone!"

This is what I needed to know a long time ago, but I am happy that with this new publication now available others will not have to suffer the way I did. Every member of an HD family and every doctor, social worker, and health professional now has an easy-to-read, exciting, yet factual tool to offer patients and their families. The quest for knowledge about Huntington's disease, as Dennis tells it, should encourage everyone to join with us and participate in the battle.

Again, Dennis clearly makes the point that our Commission for the Control of Huntington's Disease and Its Consequences did more than address HD. Our recommendations challenged scientists to study the brain and central nervous system, using HD as a prototype for genetic, psychiatric, and neurologic disorders; scientists know that research in rare disorders can sometimes unravel the mysteries of more common disorders. It is a challenge that has just begun to be met. The explosion of scientific interest and knowledge is reported in scientific journals and newspapers every day.

It is equally exciting to find out how in the clinical setting we are learning about research in the care of those who are already diagnosed with HD. Dennis originally wrote a little pamphlet because he knew that more people needed to know more about HD. This book is an outgrowth of that effort, and now we have this excellent guide to give us courage to keep going. Progress! Progress!

Marjorie Guthrie
Founder/President Emeritus CCHD, USA
Chairperson, HD Commission, USA

July 1981

Preface

In October, 1977, the Australian Broadcasting Commission televised a documentary called "Something in the Family." The program concerned a little-known and incurable hereditary disorder named Huntington's disease, which affects certain cells in the brain and often leads to gradual physical, emotional, and intellectual disintegration.

I had known about the disease before I moved from the United States to Australia in 1972. I knew, for example, that Woody Guthrie, the famous American folk singer, died with the disease in the 1960s. Viewing the documentary made me curious about what was being done in Australia to combat this unusual problem. A few days later I rang the New South Wales branch of the Australian Huntington's Disease Association. That telephone call set me on a course which eventually produced this book.

While "Something in the Family" was being shown in Australia, a concerned group of citizens and scientists in the United States were submitting to Congress a detailed, multivolume report on Huntington's disease, together with a national plan of action to do something about this and related neurological illness. During 1976–77 the United States Commission for the Control of Huntington's Disease and Its Consequences received personal testimony or written submissions from nearly 2,000 people concerned about this "rare" disorder. The accumulated testimony documented a disturbing situation. The disease was not as rare as most people believed, and many people affected either directly or indirectly by it were desperate. They felt condemned by fate, betrayed by friends, and abandoned by society. The public testimony, which was received from eleven American cities, revealed a whole catalogue of problems. Not only did the disease take a terrible toll among families, but it was poorly understood by doctors. Misdiagnosis occurred with distressing frequency, and the treatment offered sometimes did more harm than good. In addition, families with members suffering from Huntington's disease (or at risk for it) were stigmatized and discriminated against by the public, various civil authorities, insurance companies, and even hospitals and nursing homes.

After joining the Australian Huntington's Disease Association, I became increasingly aware of some of these problems. I also became familiar with the dreadful sense of hopelessness that surrounds the disease and undermines the capacity of many people to deal with it effectively. Despondency, depression, and gloom mark not just those who actually have the disease, but many otherwise healthy relatives and friends. In one way or another, every member of the family becomes a patient whose needs change with each passing year. For many, the burden becomes so great that they resign themselves to defeat very early in the struggle. The disease thus exacts a much higher toll than it would if people had a more open and positive approach and were strengthened by supportive public attitudes and institutions.

I also became concerned by the lack of comprehensive, nontechnical published information on a disease that so seriously touches the lives of many people. Most of the printed material we used in Australia was brief and derivative. We borrowed much of our information from North America or Great Britain. We could not provide affected families, general physicians, and genetic counselors with a comprehensive discussion of the many problems raised by the disorder.

In July, 1978, I received a year's leave from Macquarie University, where I teach American history. I returned to the United States to do research in my own field, but I also took time to broaden my contacts with scientists who were actively engaged in research on Huntington's disease. After discussions with a number of people, I met with Marjorie Guthrie in the New York office of the Committee to Combat Huntington's Disease. After her husband's death in 1967, Marjorie Guthrie began a crusade against Huntington's disease which has now spread around the globe. More than any other person, she is responsible for the revolution in scientific interest and public attitudes that has taken place since Woody died.

With Marjorie's encouragement, and the advice offered by various scientific and medical specialists, I decided to devote the remainder of my study leave to research for a book which would meet the needs both of affected families and of medical professionals involved in genetic counseling and in treating the disease. The main task was to translate the most useful material in technical journals into a language everyone could understand. As a person without medical training, I approached this project with some hesitation. I feared that scientists and doctors would tell me that I had no business trying to work in this field. Much to my delight, the reaction was quite the contrary. I was greeted everywhere with generous offers of assistance.

As research progressed, I became increasingly convinced that the book was vital. Families touched by Huntington's disease are hungry for detailed information on the disorder. Many turn in desperation to scientific journals. When I returned to Sydney in July, 1979, a fifteen-year-old girl approached me at one of the regular meetings of the Australian Huntington's Disease Association and asked me to help her with the meaning of the following sentence from a technical article on Huntington's disease: "Mitochondria, the rough endoplasmic reticulum, and other cytoplasmic components become sequestered into membrane-bound vesicles termed autophagic vacuoles." As I talked to this young woman, who was herself at risk for Huntington's disease, I knew that my project was on the right track.

Most of what follows in this book is written in plain, nontechnical language. I do not mean that the book is simple or easy reading. My goal has been to provide the lay reader with a comprehensive introduction to the genetic facts and clinical characteristics of Huntington's disease as well as to some of the practical and ethical problems associated with the disease. Although every attempt has been made to keep technical terminology to a minimum, the book is not intended to be simple. The subject is far too complicated and important for that. Readers who turn to a book on a subject like Huntington's disease usually have some special reason for doing so. They have more than a passing interest in the topic. These readers will have no difficulty working through the facts, problems, and concepts discussed in this book. Chapters 2 and 9 are somewhat more demanding than the rest but, even here, the attentive reader should have few problems.

The Ian Miller family discussed in chapter 1 is fictional. No such family exists, nor is the account based on the experiences of any existing family. The purpose of chapter 1 is to illustrate some of the typical symptoms of Huntington's disease and some of the problems arising when the Huntington's disease gene is present but unknown. Except for the Miller family, all persons and places named in this chapter are real. "Mary's Mount" is a functioning Huntington's disease care center in Melbourne. Dr. Edmond Chiu is involved with Huntington's disease patients through the Department of Psychiatry at the University of Melbourne, and Betty Teltscher is a social worker with extensive experience in Huntington's disease care and research. The only fictional names in this book are those given to persons and families who actually have the disease.

A book of this type is not the work of one person. I could not have completed the manuscript without the assistance and advice of many people. I am particularly indebted to those who are living with the reality of Huntington's disease and who provided extraordinary examples of courage. I hope that some of these people, along with other interested readers, will continue to offer advice and information. There may then be future, revised editions of this book. The best revisions will come from suggestions made by the readers. I welcome your ideas and criticisms. As you read this book, I hope you will make note of any criticisms or suggestions that occur to you, and mail them to me in Australia. The constructive suggestions of readers are the best response any author can receive.

I would also like to express my appreciation to the many people who have given me advice and assistance. Since this book is international in scope, perhaps acknowledgments are best made by quickly touring several nations.

In the United States I would like to thank Marjorie Guthrie, Irma Bauman, Nancy Wexler, Robert Rusk, John Pearson,

George W. Paulson, S. J. Enna, Ian Butler, Ruggero Fariello, Malcolm Stewart, Jay Pettegrew, JoAnne Tuttle, Irving Rockwood, Jane Curran Johnson, Brian Keeling, and Cory Masiak.

In Australia: David Propert, Betty Teltscher, Colin Brackenridge, Edmond Chiu, Des Brown, Robyn Kapp, Di Clifton, Don Tailby, Ron Walls, Chenya Huang, Lyn Hayes, Sheree Pearce, Stephen Reid, June Mitchell, Gwen Morris, Bruce Harris, John Kleinig, Gwen Noble, Gloria Webb, Joan Elder, Jean Scott, Chris Champion, Antony Kidman, Yvonne Fetherston, Mandy Williams, David Floate, D. C. Wallace, and Nancy Sibtain.

In Canada: T. L. Perry, André Barbeau, and F. Clarke Fraser.

In the Netherlands: George Bruyn.

Finally, I would like to thank the leaders of Huntington's disease volunteer organizations discussed in chapter 10.

Dennis Phillips

Macquarie University
New South Wales, Australia
January 1981

Living with
Huntington's
Disease

1

Huntington's Disease: What Is It?

If the Devil himself had set out to create the most cruel of diseases, he couldn't have done better than this.

Ian Miller's life had gone strangely out of control long before he realized that he had a serious health problem.[1] Until he reached the age of thirty-five, his life could have served as a textbook example of a typical Australian success story. He did well in school, became a talented athlete, and graduated with honors from the University of Melbourne. After military service in Vietnam, he returned to Australia where he married his childhood sweetheart and established a small but successful construction firm in the Melbourne suburb of Kew. He worked with the Boy Scouts, attended church regularly, and served in local government.

Ian and his wife, Jean, began a family early in their marriage. Eventually the young couple had four children, two boys and two girls. They also remained especially close to Ian's mother and his three brothers and two sisters. As the oldest of six children, and while still a teenager, Ian had become the "family patriarch" when his father died in an automobile accident. With the help of her eldest son, "Mum" Miller maintained the family and managed her modest home with dedication and skill. After Ian and Jean were married, she dearly valued their affection and help, and was especially pleased when they presented her with four handsome grandchildren.

By the mid-1970s, Ian felt on top of the world. He had a wonderful, healthy family, a spacious home, a successful business, and a promising future. He enjoyed the fellowship of a wide range of close friends. He never knew the scorn or animosity of a single enemy.

Then mysterious things began to happen. It started so vaguely that in future years Ian could not even recall the beginning of his problems. But once events began to turn against him, there seemed to be no end to them. He started to feel uneasy at about the time of his tenth wedding anniversary. Until then he had often boasted that he had never had a sick day in his life. Now he wasn't exactly "sick," but he sometimes felt that he had "a bad case of the nerves." He was restless and found that he could not sit still for long.

From week to week and month to month he experienced more and more difficulty controlling what he called "this damned nervousness." And when he became nervous, he had trouble with his temper. For years he had been a gentle and understanding husband. Now he seemed to get irritated with his wife and children at the slightest pretext. Jean scolded him for being too rough on the kids. For the first time in their married life, he shouted at her. On several occasions he hit her. She wondered if Ian had problems at work that he did not wish to discuss. She spent dark and gloomy hours worrying about what had come over him. Had she let him down somehow? Was there another woman? Had he taken to drinking secretly? There was no sign of any of it, but her husband was clearly a changed man.

Ian also realized that something was wrong, but he didn't know exactly what it was or what to do about it. He often felt depressed. When he flew into a rage at Jean or one of the children and then realized what he had done, the depression deepened. Yet he seemed unable to control his temper, his restlessness, or the bouts of depression. He knew that his life was not as happy as it had been and he believed that he was mostly to blame, but he couldn't seem to recover his old self.

He finally concluded that he was working too hard. Unfortunately, he could not afford to take time off work, because things had gone awry there too. In previous years he had managed the business very efficiently. Records were always precise and orderly.

He got along fine with the six men who worked for him, and Miller Construction had an enviable reputation throughout the city. But Ian gradually lost control. Orders were mislaid, records lost, bills forgotten. He ran into difficulties with creditors and customers alike.

For months his secretary managed to cover for him, but as the errors accumulated so too did his impatience with her. He blamed her for mistakes he knew were his own. She took it for several months, then quit. When she walked out, one of Ian's workmen spoke to Jean privately about her husband's problems on the job. Just as Jean had worried that her husband might be having trouble at work, Ian's employees assumed that their boss must be having difficulties at home. Despite everyone's concern, no one could explain the source of the problem.

It wasn't long before Ian lost some of his most reliable employees. He replaced them, but the replacements didn't last long. Soon Miller Construction began to lose its standing in the community. Nobody wanted to work for "old man Miller." But "old man" Ian Miller was only thirty-seven years old. In a few short years, he had gone from successful model citizen to a worried and detested man who faced imminent disaster both at home and on the job.

At his wife's insistence, Ian finally agreed to visit the doctor. He was told that he had a nervous condition, and mild sedatives were prescribed. When Ian received a bill for $50 for the half-hour consultation, he vowed that he would have to be carried into a hospital before he would see a doctor again.

Ian continued to believe that he did not have a serious health problem. He had developed some "nervous tics," but he believed them to be physical manifestations of the emotional stress he was under. The tics were especially obvious in his hands. Sometimes his thumb jerked involuntarily, especially when he got angry or excited. He also noticed a change in his handwriting. He found it difficult to maintain the beautiful penmanship for which he had won awards in school. He attributed it to pressures on the job and the need to write rapidly. "Look at doctors," he muttered to himself. "No one writes any worse than they do." Still, the nervousness bothered him. After a while it wasn't just his hands.

He crossed and recrossed his legs, shifted from here to there, and consciously pressed his hands together and gripped them like a vice between his knees to keep them under control.

Disappointed that her husband's visit to the doctor did not produce any improvement, Jean became more frustrated and irritated with each passing month. Finally, one weekend when Ian went into a tantrum and hit one of the children with his fist, Jean gathered all four of the kids and walked out. She moved in with her parents, who had been horrified by Ian's deteriorating conduct. Several attempts at reconciliation failed. Ian would promise to do better, then go off into one of his rages again. Eventually, Jean gave up on her marriage, sued for divorce, and won custody of the children. Ian was required by the court to pay $500 monthly in maintenance and child support just at the time when his construction firm hit rock bottom. It wasn't long before he was forced to declare bankruptcy, and shortly thereafter he fell behind in his support payments.

Ian could hardly believe what had happened. His life seemed scattered in tatters around him. He was forced to sell almost everything he owned to meet his financial obligations. He moved into a small flat in Collingwood and took whatever jobs he could find. None of them lasted long. Although he never drank heavily, he now seemed to have trouble with his balance. People accused him of being drunk when he had never taken a drink at all. He looked terrible. Moody and depressed, he saw no particular reason to take good care of himself.

Now desperate, and too ashamed to face his mother, he turned to his brothers and sisters for help. But they were unwilling to help him. They were dismayed over the way he had treated his wife and children. He had allowed his lucrative business to waste away and, worst of all, he had shown no appreciation for their advice and offers of assistance. Now they wanted nothing to do with him. They believed that anyone who didn't appreciate help didn't deserve it. Privately, they concluded that their oldest brother must have become an alcoholic, even though none of them had ever seen him drink excessively.

Rejected by his family, Ian turned to the church he had served so faithfully. He had withdrawn from the congregation several years earlier when his problems began to multiply. Now he went back in a desperate search for help. But he quickly learned that most churches are not interested in desperate people. When his marriage failed, the church gossip mills praised his wife for having the courage to leave him. Church prayer groups put his name at the top of their list, but even as his old church friends prayed for him, most of them did their best to avoid being seen with him. By being prayer-listed, he was blacklisted. When he appeared unshaven and dishevelled at a Sunday morning service, several people complained to the minister. They said no man should be allowed in God's house in such a disgraceful state. They warned that they would hold the minister personally responsible if this "dreadful episode" were ever repeated.

After the service, the minister spoke to Ian privately, offering him money if he needed help but advising him that certain standards of dress and decorum were expected of everyone who attended church. Ian accepted the money and mailed it to his children. He never attended church again.

Three days later, Ian was arrested for public drunkenness. Two policemen in a cruising patrol car spotted a man stumbling down a residential street in Collingwood. When he failed to produce identification, they drove him to the police station for booking. A breathalyzer test proved that Ian had not been drinking. He was turned over to a police lieutenant for an interview. The lieutenant happened to know Ian from previous years in Boy Scout work. He could hardly believe how much his old friend had changed. After a brief and awkward discussion of some of Ian's problems, the lieutenant handed him a card with the address of a doctor and then arranged for a car to drive him home.

Laying aside his bias against doctors, Ian made an appointment and visited the recommended physician a few days later. The physician referred him to a psychiatrist, who prescribed a sedative and recommended a long vacation. Six months later a bill collector working on behalf of both the doctor and the psychiatrist knocked on the door of Ian's flat. The place had been abandoned.

Feeling that life had lost all meaning for him, deserted by family and friends, and deeply in debt, Ian took to the road. If nothing more, it promised anonymity. When he had the money, he traveled by bus. Otherwise he hitched a ride, jumped a freight, or just walked. Nobody paid much attention to an old swaggie on the road. He traveled aimlessly—from Melbourne to Cairns and most of the way back. Finally, his mother turned to the police in an attempt to locate her son. He was picked up walking along the Pacific Highway a few miles south of Newcastle.

As a result of this and previous arrests, Ian was committed for thirty days' observation at a state psychiatric hospital in a country town. While there, he was subjected to several rounds of electric shock treatment. His condition continued to grow worse. He felt totally alone. He was too far from home to be visited by his mother, and his brothers and sisters continued to scorn him. Jean knew of his condition but, fearing for her own safety, did not venture a visit. She remained determined to protect herself and her children from this man who had changed so much. She was also angry. It had been months since Ian had made a support payment. The least he could do, she thought, was to provide for his children. She was considering taking him to court again.

During his month in the hospital, Ian's movement disorder grew markedly worse. The "nervous tics" were much more obvious and had spread to other parts of his body. Even the muscles of his face now twitched and contorted, giving him a strange, grotesque grimace. He had difficulty eating without spilling his food. Worst of all, he realized that his appearance was abhorrent to other people. When they recoiled in his presence, he tried to hide. He wanted to stay away from other people as much as he could. He became more and more depressed and withdrawn. These changes seemed to confirm the medical diagnosis that he was mentally unbalanced, but nobody could say exactly what was wrong. Doctors could come little closer to an explanation than did the nurses, who simply called him a mental case.

At the end of a month Ian was released from the hospital and returned to Melbourne in the custody of his mother, who made room for him in her home. Caring for him was a difficult task. Her other children refused to help. Instead, they urged her to send Ian back to "the loony bin." She continued to care for him at home until one day she was herself hospitalized with pneumonia. When Mum Miller went to the hospital, one of her younger sons intervened and took his oldest brother to a friend who worked in the Department of Psychiatry at the University of Melbourne. This proved to be the decisive turn because, at long last, the nature of Ian's problem was explained.

Dr. Edmond Chiu had never met Ian, but he knew much about the man's unfortunate career from conversations with Ian's younger brother. Even before seeing Ian, Dr. Chiu suspected a neurological problem. The behavioral characteristics about which Ian's brother so readily complained seemed all too familiar. How could a man stagger like a drunk when police tests proved that he had not been drinking? Why would a personality change in such a bizarre and variable manner over such a long period of time? How could Ian's physical and emotional deterioration be explained without reference to a possible organic disease? Dr. Chiu had seen many cases like this before. He suspected that a specific disease might be involved, and he had long encouraged Ian's brother to bring his troubled relative for examination.

When Ian was settled comfortably in Dr. Chiu's office, the doctor and his new patient began a detailed discussion of Ian's past. Visual observation confirmed Dr. Chiu's suspicion that Ian might be suffering from a chronic, degenerative disorder known as Huntington's disease. But since the disorder was genetic in origin, it was best diagnosed by confirming a family history which revealed the presence of the disease in previous generations. Dr. Chiu scheduled Ian for a series of neurological and psychiatric tests and then set out on his own to see if he could discover any sign of the disease in the history of the Miller family.

Dr. Chiu first visited Ian's mother, who was recuperating in a nearby city hospital. He learned from her that Ian's father had died in an automobile crash at the age of thirty-eight. Before that fatal accident, the man had been in perfect health. But Mum Miller also revealed that Ian's paternal grandmother had died in a nursing home from "a nervous condition" which everyone in the family called premature senility. When Dr. Chiu asked Mum Miller if anyone had ever mentioned Huntington's disease, she replied that she had never heard of it.

Dr. Chiu then returned to the Department of Psychiatry, where he sought the assistance of a social worker named Betty Teltscher. Among her many other duties in connection with Huntington's disease, Mrs. Teltscher served as curator of the Victorian state register on Huntington's chorea. The register had been established by Dr. Charles Brothers in the early 1950s and left to the Department of Psychiatry after his death in 1964. In addition to its confidential listing of Huntingtonian families, the register contained copies of the death certificates of people who had died with the disease. By combing through these records, Dr. Chiu and Mrs. Teltscher discovered a copy of the death certificate for Ian's grandmother. The cause of death was listed as "choking attributable to Huntington's chorea." Apparently "Nanna" Miller's doctor knew that the woman had Huntington's disease but, for reasons of his own, withheld the information from the rest of the family. A further search of the records revealed unmistakable evidence of the disease in previous generations.

With the results of Ian's tests and the Miller family history before him, Dr. Chiu discussed the case with Dr. Colin Brackenridge, Australia's most experienced researcher on the disorder. As in all their diagnoses of Huntington's disease, the two men were determined to be absolutely sure that they were not in error. Misdiagnosis of a hereditary condition as serious as Huntington's disease would be disastrous. With the information before them, they knew that they had discovered the true explanation for Ian's problems. His years of terrible suffering, his erratic behavior, the collapse of his family and business, the painful loneliness—all were due to a medical condition which had gone unrecognized until now. The next step was to explain the nature of the disease to Ian and help him come to terms with what it meant for him and his family.

Dr. Chiu scheduled a long meeting with his new patient. He began by reassuring Ian that a definitive explanation for his problems had been discovered. The doctor carefully explained that Ian was suffering from a hereditary disorder which had been in his family for many generations. The so-called premature senility from which Nanna Miller had suffered was really a genetic disease described in 1872 by an American doctor named George Huntington. The disease was traditionally called Huntington's chorea, or more recently simply Huntington's disease.[2]

Ian listened attentively as Dr. Chiu explained that the exact cause of the disease was still unknown. It is passed from one generation to the next through what is believed to be a defect in one of an individual's many genes, half of which are inherited from either parent. For this reason, any child, regardless of sex, who is born to a man or woman who carries the gene for Huntington's disease has exactly a 50 percent chance of inheriting it. Unfortunately, there is as yet no test to show who has inherited the defective gene and who has not. One can only wait until actual symptoms of the disease begin to appear, and this does not happen in most cases until the person carrying the defective gene reaches his or her late thirties or early forties. For this reason, Huntington's disease is known as a late-onset disorder.[3]

Dr. Chiu explained to Ian that in rare instances the disease appears in children. Sometimes it does not appear until the individual reaches the age of fifty, or even sixty. Anyone who has not shown any sign of the disease, but whose parent had it, can be said to be "at risk" of getting it. Everyone at risk has an exactly even chance at birth of having inherited the gene for Huntington's disease. If he has inherited it, then eventually he will show at least some signs of the disease. If he is fortunate and has not inherited the gene, there is no cause for concern, because Huntington's disease cannot hit one generation, skip over the next, and then reappear in the third or some future generation.[4]

Because Huntington's disease usually appears relatively late in life, explained Dr. Chiu, it poses some particularly difficult problems. A couple with one partner at risk for Huntington's disease must decide whether or not to have children without knowing if the disease will actually appear. If a person at risk waits until he or she is reasonably certain to be free from the defective gene before making such a decision, then it will be too late in life to have children at all.

Dr. Chiu pointed out that in Ian's case the very threat of the disease was unknown to the whole family. None of them had ever heard of Huntington's disease. The doctors Ian had visited undoubtedly knew the name of the disorder, but may never have encountered anyone who actually had it. The doctors had assumed that Ian's medical problem, if indeed there was a "medical" problem at all, was due to his personal and professional problems rather than the other way around.

Ian asked about his father. If his grandmother had the disease and it never skipped a generation, then why didn't his father show any sign of it? Dr. Chiu explained that, since Huntington's disease had been confirmed in Ian's paternal grandmother and in Ian himself, it was now clear that his father had also carried the defective gene but had died in the automobile accident before symptoms of the disease became apparent. This was quite conceivable, since the accident occurred when Ian's father was still relatively young. If he had lived long enough, there was no doubt that he too would have shown signs of the disorder eventually. Even though he never demonstrated overt symptoms, he carried the gene, and *each* of his children was at 50 percent risk of having inherited it.

Ian listened to Dr. Chiu's explanation and understood. His eyes filled with tears, not so much for himself, but for what this meant for his brothers and sisters and for his own children. Ian now had ten nieces and nephews, all on his side of the family because his wife was an only child. Dr. Chiu calculated that there were nineteen people in the Miller family who were actually or potentially at risk for Huntington's disease. As yet, not one of them knew that such a disease existed. Dr. Chiu reviewed the situation: Ian's three brothers and two sisters, as well as his own four children, were all at 50 percent risk. His ten nieces and nephews were potentially at risk, depending on whether or not their respective parents carried the gene for the disorder.

As Ian grappled with the implications of this news, he grew angry. He told Dr. Chiu that if the Devil himself had set out to create the most cruel of diseases, he couldn't have done better than this. Who was to tell his family about the presence of this dreadful hereditary condition? How would his brothers and sisters react when they learned that each of them had a fifty-fifty chance of getting the disease that had caused the behavior they so detested in their oldest brother? What about his own children? Ian was particularly shaken when he realized that he had passed the risk of the disease to his children without even knowing what he was doing. Dr. Chiu cautioned Ian that he must not blame himself for things over which he had no control. But Ian wondered aloud whether he would have made a different decision on marriage and a family if he had known about Huntington's disease from an early age.

Dr. Chiu watched Ian closely for signs of fatigue, but his new friend was filled with questions about the disease and about the future. Was there a cure? How about treatment? Could the condition be reversed or at least halted? What did the future hold for someone who had Huntington's disease? Dr. Chiu explained that generalizations are difficult to make because no two cases of the disease are exactly the same. Some people manage for years with only minor difficulties. Others are completely incapacitated. In some people the disease progresses rapidly, but in others it is not so serious and takes a much slower course.

Placing a reassuring hand on Ian's shoulder, Dr. Chiu explained that Huntington's disease is characterized by a gradual destruction of certain brain cells. Once that process begins, it cannot be reversed. Some cells in the body regenerate, but this is not true of brain cells. Since scientists do not as yet know what precise mechanism triggers the deterioration in the brain, there is no complete explanation for the disease and no cure.

On the other hand, recent advances in drug therapy have made possible more effective control of the disorder. The involuntary muscle movements can be checked in many cases, and drugs are also used to combat the emotional problems often associated with the disease. Unfortunately, little can be done to reverse the intellectual impairment, or dementia, which is sometimes associated with the disorder. Dr. Chiu emphasized that symptoms vary significantly from one patient to the next. Some people have major problems with chorea, or involuntary muscle movement, but relatively little emotional imbalance or intellectual deterioration. But the condition, whatever form it takes, is progressive. Once it begins, it cannot be reversed. Most Huntington's disease patients face fifteen to twenty years of gradual decline until death.[5]

Dr. Chiu pieced the facts together slowly so that Ian would have time to absorb them. This was a heavy burden for anyone to assume in such a short time, especially a man who had been through so much in recent years. But Ian was interested and resilient. Even though he suffered to some extent from all three major aspects of the disease—involuntary movements, emotional disturbance, and occasional intellectual problems—he was fully capable of comprehending all that Dr. Chiu told him. The doctor congratulated Ian on his tough and positive attitude, and remarked that such an attitude would be very important in the future.

During the conversation, Dr. Chiu questioned Ian to assure that everything was understood correctly. Errors were carefully corrected. For example, Ian erroneously concluded that, since he had four children and Huntington's disease had a 50 percent risk factor, two of the four would inherit the disease and two would not. He wanted to know which two were most likely to inherit the disease. Would it be the oldest? . . . the youngest? . . . the two boys? . . . the two girls? Dr. Chiu quickly explained that the 50 percent risk did *not* mean that exactly half of Ian's children would get the disease and half would be free from it. All the 50 percent risk meant was that each individual child had at birth an exactly even chance of inheriting the disorder.

Dr. Chiu pointed out that the process is random—somewhat similar to the flip of a coin. If you flip a coin four times, he explained, you may or may not get two heads and two tails. The combination may be four heads and no tails, or one head and three tails, etc. But if you flip a coin many times, the average of heads and tails will be about equal. So it is with Huntington's disease. All the children of a Huntington's disease carrier may inherit the disease, or half of them, or one, or none. What can be said with accuracy is that *each* of them faces an exactly even chance. Theoretically, it was possible that all the other members of the Miller family would be fortunate enough to escape the disease. However, with a risk factor so high, it was much more likely that other members of the family also carried the defective gene and would eventually manifest symptoms similar to those Ian now experienced. Only time would tell who that might be.

With Ian beginning to show signs of fatigue, Dr. Chiu arranged for him to be driven home. The two men made an appointment to meet every day for the next week. During these meetings they reviewed some of the major events in Ian's life and interpreted them in terms of the classic early symptoms of Huntington's disease. Some of the earliest signs were so subtle that they became obvious only in retrospect. Dr. Chiu pointed out that this is why the initial diagnosis of Huntington's disease can be so difficult, especially in the absence of a family history confirming the presence of the disorder. Early behavioral symptoms may be so slight that they are indistinguishable from what would be considered normal in anyone not known to be at risk for the disease.[6] This was true in Ian's case, in which the earliest signs took the form of excessive "nervousness" and some emotional instability. These early signals were so subtle that even if Ian had known about Huntington's disease he might not have been able to identify its presence.

Dr. Chiu explained that the early signs may appear in any or all of three areas—physical, emotional, and intellectual.[7] The first physical (motor) symptoms may be fidgeting, a twitching in the thumb or fingers, or excessive restlessness. There may be clumsiness, alterations in handwriting, or difficulty with normal daily physical skills such as driving. Ian recounted early experiences with some of these problems. Dr. Chiu remarked that these initial symptoms usually become more pronounced with time. They develop into involuntary jerks and twitches of the head, neck, arms, and legs. Ian was well aware that his movement problems had increased over the months and years. Dr. Chiu now had him on some medicine that calmed him down and made the movements much less severe.

Dr. Chiu went on to explain that when chorea is present the movements usually increase during periods of voluntary effort, stress, or excitement, and diminish during rest, often disappearing entirely when the patient is asleep. In advanced cases, the constant involuntary physical activity during waking hours may result in a ravenous appetite with a simultaneous loss of weight. Ian recalled that he had lost more than thirty pounds during the last year, a loss which he had attributed to worry.[8]

When the muscles of the face, tongue, and mouth become involved, Dr. Chiu continued, the person may have difficulty speaking, eating, and swallowing. Coupled with emotional disturbances and intellectual deterioration, these advanced symptoms represent Huntington's disease at its worst. Because these patients become "unattractive," many "normal" people are upset by them and may seek to avoid or isolate them. The patients are aware of this and become ashamed. Frequently, the problems associated with Huntington's disease become very much worse due to a patient's isolation and the frustration and embarrassment he feels about his condition. The more attention, communication, support, and love the person receives at all stages of the disorder, the greater are his chances of coping with it effectively.[9] Ian thought about his own brothers and sisters. He no longer blamed them for their disdain. They had no way of knowing that he was sick and not just mean.

Late in the week, Dr. Chiu met Ian at the University Unit at Parkville near the Royal Melbourne Zoo. The two men toured the zoo, walked the fringes of a nearby public golf course, and then returned to the gardens of the Parkville center. Some patients from the center were soaking up the warm sun in the gardens. As the two men walked past row after row of flowers, Dr. Chiu commented on other aspects of Huntington's disease.

In addition to the initial physical symptoms, there are sometimes subtle intellectual signs as well. These may involve little more than a slightly reduced ability to organize routine matters or cope effectively with novel situations. There might be a loss of recent memory. Business activities could become more difficult than usual. Ian told Dr. Chiu about the way the construction firm had slipped from his control. He mentioned the forgotten bills, the lost records, the orders that were never filled. Now he seemed to have less trouble with that sort of thing, but now he had no job and few responsibilities.

Dr. Chiu explained that in addition to the physical and intellectual symptoms, there could be emotional signs as well. These might take the form of an accentuation of certain aspects of the individual's normal behavior—bouts of depression, periods of apathy, various forms of impulsiveness, or even violence. Personality changes occur. The person might become especially irritable or lose interest in personal appearance and hygiene. There might be periods of confusion or bizarre behavior. Relatives and friends might ask what had "come over" the individual to make him change so much.[10]

The two men paused briefly to exchange greetings with a man tending a large bed of beautiful yellow and red roses. Ian suspected immediately that this man also had Huntington's disease, and Dr. Chiu later confirmed this. As they moved through the garden, Dr. Chiu asked Ian's opinion on the design of a nearby greenhouse where other patients were at work. Ian said he was no expert on greenhouses, but he judged that this one could stand some improvement. Dr. Chiu nodded a thoughtful agreement.

During the drive back to Ian's flat, Dr. Chiu explained that one of the worst aspects of Huntington's disease is the level of public ignorance about it and related disorders. An undeserved stigma is often placed on people who have chronic, degenerative illnesses. A society that puts so much emphasis on youth, good health, and physical beauty is bound to neglect the elderly and the sick. Discrimination has become a fact of life for sufferers of serious, debilitating diseases. Society is not meeting the needs of people who suffer from these diseases. Even persons who are *at risk* for Huntington's disease are discriminated against. It is difficult for them to obtain insurance; they sometimes suffer at the hands of employers; they are often viewed with suspicion or pity by friends; and governments treat them as if they were nothing more than a potential social burden. Huntington's disease has been aptly described as a " 'downwardly mobile' disease fraught with fear, shame, guilt, and an overwhelming financial burden."[11]

When the two men met again in Dr. Chiu's office, Ian was invited to listen to some authentic case histories that revealed how other people had faced the challenge of living with Huntington's disease. Dr. Chiu removed from a shelf a large, paperback volume. He explained that this book, and similar volumes still on the shelf, contained public testimony offered to the United States Commission for the Control of Huntington's Disease and Its Consequences. He opened the volume, which contained testimony taken in Texas in 1977, and asked Ian to read a copy of an anonymous letter addressed from Houston.

> It is with great trauma that I attempt to put into words the story of my life with a mother who had Huntington's chorea. . . . When I was in junior high school, my mother was as normal as I can remember her ever being. . . . By the time I was in high school, life was a nightmare for me. Mother switched between being euphoric and volatile, and I never knew what to expect.
> By the time I was in college . . . Mother had less control over her extremities. She acted as if she had St. Vitus' Dance. She had several operations during this period of her life, and the doctors never referred to her emotional state or strange be-

havior. This only confirmed in my mind, that Mother was just a nervous wreck. My father used the 'head-in-the-sand' approach to her in order to survive. . . .

At one point, Mother went to the dental school to see about her teeth. She sat all day long, and no one would help her. . . . Finally, after six hours, one dentist told her to go home . . . and advised her to see a psychiatrist.

When Mother was in her early sixties, she backed into a space heater and burned 50 percent of her body. Daddy called me three days later and thought she needed to see a doctor! He would not take her. In the middle of the night, a doctor and I went to see her. . . . A neurologist was called in, and, after extensive tests, told me that Mother was in the advanced stages of a disease I had never heard of—Huntington's chorea. . . .

Mother underwent extensive skin graftings in the hospital for six weeks. At the end of that time, the surgeon told me I could take her home, and I panicked. I felt that care at home was totally out of the question, for Daddy would not help. I then looked at or called 43 nursing homes to see who could take her on what we could afford to pay. We found one, and she stayed there for six months. I found out later that they had controlled her by giving her four times the amount of Thorazine prescribed by the doctor!

She was taken to Austin in an ambulance, strapped down, with no stops along the way. . . . The next phase is nightmare number 1000. From the time Mother was admitted into the hospital, her social worker tried to get her out! . . . They tried to send her home on "furlough" for Christmas, stating she could stay with me for a month. I immediately let them know that in no way was this possible, for Mother or for me. . . .

Then . . . a claims adjuster sent me a letter, stating that I owed the hospital $11,000 for back payment . . . my father and I sold his home, he moved in with me, and we gave the hospital what they asked for. . . . The hospital moved Mother within a year to a nursing home in Austin, where she remained for three years until she died.

My age is 48. . . . My husband and several doctors have strongly advised against my telling my three children (ages 18, 22, and 24) about Huntington's chorea being in the family and letting them know their risks. . . .[12]

Ian shook his head in disbelief. It was hard to accept the fact that a single disease could do so much damage. Dr. Chiu observed that the letter illustrated many of the tragedies associated with Huntington's disease. But then he asked Ian to compare what he had just read to another letter written by a woman in Waco, Texas.

My husband is a patient at [a local hospital] here in Waco, Texas. . . . When we married 31 years ago I knew that my husband was a potential victim, as his mother was affected and several members of her immediate family. I studied all I could concerning the disease and still chose to marry. So you see, when my husband did show signs of Huntington's, this came as no surprise. I had more or less conditioned myself to meet all of the social, financial, etc. situations that would come my way.

Ed and I also chose to have children. . . . We told our children about the disease and the chances of them having it and we feel that they have accepted it and are learning to live with it as we did and are. We have left the decision of whether they will have children to them. We have told them that before they go into marriage that they should tell the person about the disease.

We haven't encountered as many problems as some of my husband's relatives have. . . . I do know that it has caused divorces, suicide and extreme financial problems in some cases.

My husband and I were 21 when we married and the first symptoms appeared when Ed was 36. His first signs were his coordination and balance. However, we feel the key to the whole thing is staying busy and being productive . . . making a victim feel he is still useful. Ed was able to work full-time until he was 48. That is not to say that we didn't have problems and some disappointments. I am convinced that he was fired from two different jobs because of his jerkiness but, of course, the employer would not give this as a reason.

This was very demoralizing and wounding to the ego but with great faith and love we were able to overcome this.

. . . Because Ed was a veteran I was able to avail the services of the veterans' hospital, but to those victims who are not veterans, there is very little available to them. . . . No doctor ever diagnosed Ed's illness. On the contrary, we told them what he had. It was only the last four years that we told even close friends about Ed's illness because there was so much stigma attached. . . .[13]

Dr. Chiu closed the book and returned it to the shelf. He gave Ian a few minutes to mull over what he had read. Then the doctor talked about the two letters. He pointed out that there were important lessons to be learned by comparing them. Obviously the woman from Waco had been able to cope with the situation better than the woman in Houston. There were several reasons for this: first, the woman from Waco was not herself at risk; second, she was able to rely upon a government-supported health facility (a Veterans Administration hospital) which was not available to the mother of the woman in Houston; third, she was strengthened by a deep commitment to her husband; finally, and perhaps most important, from the very beginning she was informed about Huntington's disease and knew what could possibly happen. The disease held no hidden terrors for her.

As Ian expressed an interest in this comparison, Dr. Chiu prepared some coffee. He served Ian's coffee in a cup especially designed for people with involuntary motor movements to allow them to handle it comfortably without spilling the contents. Then Dr. Chiu elaborated on the four points of comparison he had just made.

He pointed out that the first letter unintentionally reflected as much concern for its author as it did for the author's mother. The letter is not only about a mother who had Huntington's disease but, more particularly, about "*my life* with a mother" who had the disease. Dr. Chiu observed that children living at risk often see in already affected parents an image of what they themselves could become. They must cope not only with a seriously ill parent, but also with their own fears. That is a lot to ask of anyone, he noted. In this particular case, the situation was made much worse by ignorance. The family did not even know what they were dealing with until the woman's mother was in the advanced stages of the disease. If the daughter's account of her father's actions was accurate, it seemed clear that he was incapable of helping. Even though only one person in the family actually suffered from the disease, everyone's life was changed as a result of its presence.

Dr. Chiu praised Ed's wife, who knew that "the key to the whole thing is staying busy and being productive." The doctor reminded Ian that most people are far more capable of living with the disease than is generally recognized. An enormous amount of work remains to be done to provide recreational and occupational therapy opportunities for patients with Huntington's disease. Too often these patients are abandoned by their families and by a society that wants nothing to do with them. A person whom everyone else gives up on is likely to give up on himself. Some healthy people, including those who work in hospitals and should know better, use unfortunate terms like "a basket case." They park the so-called basket case in an isolated corner of a mental institution, hospital, or nursing home and try to forget it. That is not a very creative way to deal with any disease.[14]

Ian remarked that Ed and his wife had coped effectively with what was a very great challenge. Dr. Chiu agreed, emphasizing that both Ed and his wife were well informed about the reality of their situation. They did not try to deny or escape it. They knew about the disease, recognized the risk, prepared themselves as much as possible for all eventualities, and shared the facts with their children. People who learn the truth about Huntington's disease at a reasonably early age are usually more capable of coping with it effectively than those who remain unaware.[15] Dr. Chiu noted that the children of the woman who wrote the first letter might well escape the disease, but they certainly should have been told that the disorder was in the family. They were entitled to the information when making their own major decisions in life. Furthermore, a knowledge of the disease would help them to better understand and assist both their grandmother and their mother. Hereditary diseases do not just go away because people prefer to ignore or deny them.

When Ian next visited Dr. Chiu's office, he found that the doctor was not alone. Dr. Chiu introduced Ian to David Propert, a geneticist and Huntington's disease researcher at the Royal Melbourne Institute of Technology. David told Ian that he had a surprise for him, and led the way to a car parked just outside Dr. Chiu's office.

As the two men drove through Melbourne's attractive suburbs, David explained their mission: "Ian, I want to show you a place called Mary's Mount. It is a splendid estate built by a man named Oliver Gilpin in the early 1930s. The buildings were constructed in the old tradition and are as solid as the houses built by Miller

Construction Company." Ian smiled at this generous reference to his old business.

"Gilpin himself never made much use of it," continued David. "It was purchased in 1945 by the Missionary Sisters of the Sacred Heart who named it Mary's Mount. That was a good name, because it occupies the second highest position in the whole city and commands a breathtaking view, especially at night, when the lights of the city shine like a jewel at its feet. The sisters eventually decided that the estate was too much for them to handle, and in 1978 they put it up for auction. In the meantime, three groups had come together in an effort to secure a site for a specialized care center for people with Huntington's disease. As a result of a 1977 Australian Broadcasting Commission television documentary, the Wesley Central Mission was alerted to the needs of persons touched by the disorder. The mission combined its resources with those of the Australian Huntington's Disease Association[16] and the University of Melbourne's Department of Psychiatry and went looking for a suitable site. After months of searching, they bought Mary's Mount in October, 1978, for $755,000. They then put another $500,000 into improving the place, and you are about to see the results."

David wheeled his car off Whitehorse Road onto a side street which intersected with Yarrbat Avenue in the suburb of Balwyn. Then he turned left through a gate in a high, red wooden fence. The car moved slowly up a long drive toward an imposing two-storey mansion. To the left of the driveway rose towering eucalyptus trees. Exotic plants spilled over the edges of peaceful ponds, which were set among stone walkways and arched bridges. The driveway led past a lawn and a spacious rose garden to the front of the mansion. Next to the central residence were a number of satellite buildings which Ian later learned served as dormitories and recreational halls.

Leaving the car, the two men walked up the wide, semicircular steps to the front door of the main building. Inside, people were busy in an office and library to the left side of the entrance and in conversation and recreation rooms to the right. Huntington's disease patients could be seen everywhere. Some were working outside in the rose garden, others were listening to music inside, and still others were helping to arrange tables for lunch. In one room a music therapist led several people in a group sing around an old piano. Ian didn't think they sounded very good at all, but that didn't matter. What mattered was that these people were *singing!*

As they toured Mary's Mount, David explained that the whole estate was devoted exclusively to the care of Huntington's disease patients. The patients with advanced symptoms were upstairs; those with more moderate disabilities were on the ground floor where they could come and go with ease; and some who were self-supporting lived in adjacent dormitories. Others were out-patients who came to Mary's Mount during the day and returned to their own homes in the suburbs late in the afternoon. Mary's Mount had a small bus, manned by volunteer drivers, to collect day patients in the morning and return them to their homes in the afternoon. "The whole idea," David explained, "is to give every-one a chance to keep busy and contribute as much as possible. I don't think there is a place in the world quite like this."

The two men toured the buildings, walked around the ponds, then arrived at the rose garden. "As you can see," said David, "the grounds here are enormous and require much care. We know about your construction experience, and I understand you have a good eye for landscaping too. Remember when Dr. Chiu asked you about that greenhouse at Parkville? Well, he had something in mind. We need a man of your background here at Mary's Mount. We have a groundskeeper who supervises the work, and he has been talking about building a new greenhouse down by the ponds. He could certainly use your advice. He could also use your help taking care of all these roses." David indicated the expanse of rose bushes with a sweep of his hand. "If you ever get to feeling that any of it is too much for you, then there is plenty of activity inside the main house. We can't offer you much other than room and board and a small salary, but it is a steady and worth-while job. Are you willing to take it on?"

A few days later David's car appeared again in front of Dr. Chiu's office. Ian and Dr. Chiu were waiting with all Ian's belongings packed into a single suitcase that David had loaned him for the occasion. Ian shook the doctor's hand and thanked him for all he had done. Dr. Chiu told his patient that he often visited Mary's Mount, and looked forward to seeing the improvement Ian would make in the roses. Ian smiled and stepped into the car. He and David soon fell into talk about greenhouse construction.

Dr. Chiu watched until the car disappeared into commuter traffic. Returning to his office, he made some coffee and slumped thoughtfully into a deep chair. He was happy that Ian now had a brighter, more hopeful future. But that was not enough. The medical condition that had changed Ian's life was not just an individual problem. It was a family disorder. Now Dr. Chiu had to turn his attention to the task of informing nineteen of Ian's relatives, none of whom had any idea that their own future might be clouded by something called Huntington's disease.

2

Huntington's Disease:
What Causes It?

*It would take a book of encyclopedia size to write my personal
stories of suffering, anxiety, poverty and desperation caused
by Huntington's disease. . . . Please! Please! Do
something now!*

The preceding account illustrates some of the medical and social
problems that are often associated with Huntington's disease.
We turn now to a very different sort of question: what *causes*
Huntington's disease? The shortest and most accurate answer,
regrettably, is that no one knows. It is generally believed, however, that Huntington's disease (HD) is caused by a defective gene
on one of the autosomes, or nonsex chromosomes. This is why
Huntington's disease is clinically defined as an "*autosomal* dominant, neurological disorder." In this chapter we will investigate
more exactly what that means.

To understand the nature of an illness like Huntington's
disease, it is important to know something about heredity and
genetics. Readers who have studied biology or life sciences in
school will probably recall that the science of modern genetics was
founded in the 1860s by a Moravian monk named Gregor Mendel.
At the heart of Mendel's work was the discovery that hereditary
traits were determined by elementary units transmitted from one
generation to the next in uniform and predictable fashion. During
Mendel's time it was commonly believed that the characteristics
of the parents were *blended* together in the children, much as one

might blend two liquids by mixing them in a single container. Traces of this misconception survive in expressions like "mixed blood" and "full blood." Mendel demonstrated in his plant-breeding experiments that there is no mixing or blending. Rather, inherited characteristics are carried by tiny particles which we now call genes.[1]

Genes are very small. The human body is composed of about 100 *trillion* cells, *each* of which contains a full complement of genes. One author has described the study of genetics as "an inward voyage of exploration" toward a goal that becomes ever more minute.[2] Not only do we travel inward into smaller and smaller particles—the cell, the nucleus of the cell, chromosomes, genes—but the more we progress the more we appreciate how far we may yet have to go. As each objective is reached, a new one appears beyond it.

Over the years, many scientists built upon the foundations laid down by Gregor Mendel. The correspondence between Mendel's hereditary units (which he called "characters") and genes contained in chromosomes was first demonstrated by Thomas Hunt Morgan at Columbia University. All living organisms have chromosomes, which are coiled, threadlike structures abiding in the heart of the cells. Arranged about the chromosomes, rather like beads strung upon a thread, are many minute particles. These are the genes. The gene is now known to be the basic unit of heredity and the source of every trait in an organism.

Genes are themselves made of a substance called DNA (deoxyribonucleic acid). The traditional model for DNA looks something like the rungs and sides of a rope ladder which has been twisted around itself. In 1953–54 two scientists, Francis H. Crick and James D. Watson, unraveled the mystery of the molecular structure of that twisted rope ladder. The arrangement of elements (called nucleotides) on the DNA ladder is itself an essential part of the instructions needed to produce every characteristic in the developing organism. The genetic orders go out to every living thing, from the tiniest bacterium to the largest whale. Human beings are subject to the same fundamental biochemical process.

The number of genes and possible combinations of genes is enormous. A single human cell may contain hundreds of thousands, perhaps millions, of genes.[3] It should come as no surprise, then, that discovering the source of a genetic disorder—a task that may involve tracking down a single gene—is not easy.

The person reading this book, like everyone who has ever lived, began life not as a combination of millions of cells but as a single cell only a few thousandths of an inch in diameter. At the moment the female egg was fertilized by the male sperm, the genetic blueprint was present which would determine the full complement of individual characteristics in the new human being. Half of the necessary chromosomes come from the father and half from the mother. In 1956 J. H. Tjio and Albert Levan at the University of Lund in Sweden demonstrated that there are forty-six chromosomes in human cells. The forty-six chromosomes (each containing many genes) are arranged in twenty-three pairs. Twenty-two of the pairs are composed of two similar chromosomes known as autosomes, or nonsex chromosomes. The other pair are the sex chromosomes.

This arrangement of chromosomes by pairs poses an interesting question. What prevents both halves of the pair from being expressed? For example, when two genes, one for blue eyes and one for brown eyes, are present, why doesn't a child have eyes that are a mix of blue and brown, or else one blue eye and one brown eye? Mendel's original plant experiments provided the answer to this problem. He discovered that each hereditary trait is the result of the interaction of two factors (called alleles) working as a pair. Since both factors cannot be expressed simultaneously, one tends to *dominate* or mask the other. Mendel learned, for example, that in flowers the allele for redness dominates that for whiteness, and the allele for round seeds dominates that for wrinkled seeds. The weaker factor is said to be recessive. A recessive factor is always masked in the presence of a dominant factor. Under the right circumstances—when two recessive alleles are coupled—a recessive characteristic is expressed. In human beings, as in other organisms, there are dominant and recessive factors. Black hair is dominant, blond hair is recessive; brown eyes, dominant, blue eyes, recessive.

The structure and function of a human being depend on such complex and myriad biochemical combinations that it would be remarkable enough if only a few of us turned out satisfactorily.

The marvel is that the system works consistently well. Very few of us end up with our toes on our hands or our ears on our knees. But the genetic mechanism is very complex, and sometimes things do go wrong. When this happens, it is usually one of three broad problems: (1) chromosomal abnormalities, (2) single gene (Mendelian) defects, and (3) polygenic disorders, involving a combination of genes.[4] Huntington's disease is believed to be a single gene defect. Before turning to an examination of this class of disorders, however, let us consider some of the problems which may arise when alterations occur in the basic chromosomal structure.

CHROMOSOMAL ABNORMALITIES

One of the most familiar examples of chromosomal abnormalities is Down's syndrome, or mongolism. In 1959 the French physician Jerome Lejeuné and his colleagues proved that this neurological disorder, characterized by Mongoloid appearance and mental retardation, is usually associated with a chromosome count of forty-seven rather than the normal forty-six. The affected individual is born with an extra number-21 chromosome (called trisomy 21). This is what causes the disease.[5]

Down's syndrome is not the only instance of an extra chromosome producing serious consequences. The phenomenon may appear with any other chromosome. The result is often mental retardation, malformations of certain parts of the body, and other abnormalities. For reasons which are not yet completely understood, Down's syndrome and other chromosome-related birth defects are more likely to occur when the mother is past the age of thirty-five.[6]

Among the many other conditions caused by chromosomal abnormalities are some involving the sex chromosomes. For example, males with an extra X (female sex) chromosome mature with a sex chromosome pattern of XXY rather than the normal XY. This condition, called Klinefelter's syndrome, is marked by both physical and psychological problems related to sex determination and expression.[7]

Just as males may have an extra X chromosome, females may

be born with a missing X chromosome (XO rather than the normal XX). If this happens, the ovaries are underdeveloped and the woman can rarely produce children of her own. The condition, known as Turner's syndrome, is one of the most common abnormalities leading to spontaneous abortion. Only about 2 percent of Turner's syndrome conceptions are carried to term and result in a live birth.[8]

The spontaneous abortions associated with Turner's syndrome illustrate how the body sometimes senses that something is wrong and rids itself of an abnormal fetus. Despite these self-cleansing mechanisms, however, live births with chromosomal abnormalities are not rare. About one in every 200 live births involves a significant chromosomal problem. Twenty thousand babies with chromosomal abnormalities are born every year in the United States alone. Fortunately, most recognized chromosomal abnormalities can be diagnosed in the fetus. With the foreknowledge that their baby will be born with a serious disability, the parents can at least consider the option of terminating the pregnancy.[9]

RECESSIVE GENETIC DISORDERS

As previously noted, a recessive gene is any gene whose expression is submerged in the presence of a dominant gene. Alternative genes for the same trait are called alleles, and recessive characteristics only become apparent when the individual inherits two recessive alleles.[10] Inheritance of a recessive allele that happens to be associated with a disorder will not necessarily produce the disorder. Persons who have inherited a normal allele with the defective allele may remain healthy if the normal allele is dominant over the defective, recessive allele. These people are carriers of the recessive disorder, but they do not themselves show symptoms of it. The defect will only become apparent when there is no dominant normal allele present. When is this likely to happen?

The probability that a recessive disorder will occur is easily illustrated by a simple block diagram. Let us suppose that two healthy carriers of a recessive disease marry and have children. The capital letter A represents the healthy allele and the small a

the defective allele. Both parents are carriers (*Aa*), but neither shows symptoms of the disease because the recessive trait is masked by the dominant allele. What is the likely result? Statistically, one-fourth of the children from this marriage could be expected to inherit a "double dose" of the defective gene and express the recessive disease. The disorder manifests itself only when both alleles (*aa*) for the condition are present.[11]

Normal (Carrier) Parent = *Aa* ↓	*A*	*a*	Normal (Carrier) ← Parent = *Aa*
A	*AA* (Normal)	*Aa* (Carrier)	
a	*Aa* (Carrier)	*aa* (Affected)	

Figure 2.1. Inheritance pattern for recessive genetic conditions. From A. E. H. Emery, *Elements of Medical Genetics*, 4th ed. (Berkeley: University of California Press, 1975).

Some recessive genetic conditions are well known. They may or may not be sex-linked, depending on whether the defective gene is located on one of the sex chromosomes. Hemophilia, or "bleeding disease," is a familiar example caused by recessive genes located on one of the female's sex (X) chromosomes. The disease occurs because the body fails to produce a functional protein called factor VIII which is required to make the blood clot properly.

Queen Victoria was one of history's most famous carriers of the recessive trait for hemophilia. It spread from her to other crowned heads of Europe, with Victoria's female descendants acting as carriers and some of her less fortunate male descendants manifesting the disease. For example, Victoria's granddaughter Alexandra, who was a carrier, married Czar Nicholas II of Russia. Their only son and heir, Alexis, was a hemophiliac. Some historians theorize that had Alexis been healthy the Russian Revolution might never have happened, at least not when it did.[12]

Hemophilia is a sex-linked recessive disorder. There are also recessive defects associated with the autosomes (nonsex chromosomes). Tay-Sachs disease is one particularly cruel example. Most Tay-Sachs babies appear quite normal at birth. But after a few months, they begin to show telltale signs of physical weakness. Rather than grow stronger like normal babies, they become weaker until they can no longer sit without support. They lose their ability to focus their eyes and become acutely sensitive to noise. As the condition gradually worsens, Tay-Sachs babies become blind and paralyzed, unable to move or eat. Few survive past the age of three or four years. In the 1960s, between 100 and 200 of these children were born every year in the United States.[13]

This condition was first described in the nineteenth century by Warren Tay, a British eye doctor, and Bernard Sachs, an American neurologist. Dr. Sachs observed that most victims of the disease were children of Ashkenazic Jews from eastern Europe. Only about 15 percent of children with Tay-Sachs disease are not Jewish. Eventually it was discovered that about one in every thirty Ashkenazic Jews carries the recessive gene for Tay-Sachs. The disease appears only when both parents are carriers. Every child of such a union has one chance in four of having Tay-Sachs.

Until recently nothing could be done about Tay-Sachs disease. In 1969 Drs. John O'Brien and Shintaro Okada of the University of California at San Diego discovered that children with Tay-Sachs disease lack an essential enzyme (hexosaminidase A, or "hex A") which prevents fatty substances called sphingolipids from accumulating in the brain. It is the gradual accumulation of these fatty substances in the brain of Tay-Sachs babies that leads to the progressive symptoms of the disease. Since hex A is normally found in the amniotic fluid surrounding the fetus, Tay-Sachs is among the many conditions that can be detected by prenatal testing.[14]

Another recessive condition, phenylketonuria, or PKU, provides an excellent example of the successful struggle to understand and manage difficult genetic disorders. There is reason to hope that Huntington's disease—provided it continues to receive the intensive research attention it deserves—may one day be managed as successfully as PKU is now.

The PKU story begins in 1934 when a Norwegian doctor, Ashborn Følling, discovered that the urine of certain mentally retarded children turned green when a chemical called ferric chloride was added. The green color was caused by the presence of a molecule known as phenylpyruvic acid which is not normally present in the urine. Scientists later demonstrated that phenylpyruvic acid and a number of other abnormal metabolites of the amino acid phenylalanine were excreted in the urine in PKU due to the deficiency in the liver of a specific enzyme that normally oxidizes phenylalanine to the related amino acid tyrosine. This enzyme is deficient because of an abnormal, autosomal recessive gene. Consequently, PKU is inherited according to the usual pattern of recessive genetic disorders.[15]

Researchers investigating PKU guessed that the condition might be controlled by adjusting the diet of affected children. In trials, infants were put on a special diet low in phenylalanine, the amino acid from which phenylpyruvic acid and related substances are formed. The diet may have been unappetizing, but its result was spectacular: it prevented the mental retardation associated with PKU.

Development of a special diet, however, did not by itself solve the problem. Since the diet must be started when the child is very young, how were doctors to determine if the newborn infant had PKU? The incidence of the disease in the United States is only about one in every 10,000 births. But that one is obviously worth saving. A simple, accurate, but reasonably inexpensive screening test was needed. In 1961 Dr. Robert Guthrie reported from Buffalo, New York, that such a test had been perfected.

Basically, the test works like this: A small sample of blood is taken from the baby's heel a few days after birth. It is cultured for eighteen hours in a specifically prepared colony of bacteria. By checking for bacterial growth, medical technicians can tell at a glance if the infant's test shows any sign of the presence of PKU. In the vast majority of cases, the test result is negative. For the minority of positive tests, more refined analysis can confirm whether PKU is actually present.

The test proved so effective that massive PKU screening and treatment programs were soon begun in many countries throughout the world. Today, the U.S. screening program detects about 200 PKU babies each year. These infants are placed on a closely monitored diet. In most cases, the diet can be moderated or discontinued entirely when the child reaches the age of six or seven years.[16]

The improvements noted in PKU babies had important implications for the struggle against other genetic diseases. William L. Nyhan, chairman of the Department of Pediatrics at the University of California, summarized the wider significance of PKU research and control: "These results represented a major breakthrough in the treatment of genetic disease. It is one that has provided hope for the treatment of other forms of mental retardation and of genetic disease in general."[17]

There are many important differences, however, between PKU and Huntington's disease, even though both are disorders which involve the death of brain cells. PKU research has not led to any breakthrough in the search for the ultimate explanation of HD. It is certainly conceivable that when the root cause of HD is finally discovered some dietary function may be involved. It is also possible, of course, that diet is not a significant aspect of the HD picture. At this stage, we simply do not know. The point is that the PKU story provides an excellent example of how a disease considered hopeless only twenty-five years ago is now detected and treated with amazing success. This type of victory serves as the basis for a cautiously optimistic approach to Huntington's disease.

DOMINANT GENETIC DISORDERS

Disorders like PKU, Tay-Sachs disease, and hemophilia are the result of recessive genetic defects. When the flawed gene happens to be dominant, the risk of recurrence is much higher. Why is this so?

Another block diagram illustrates how dominant genetic conditions differ from recessive disorders. One parent (*Aa*) carries the HD gene. Since HD is a late-onset disorder, this parent may not yet know that he or she has the gene and will eventually develop symptoms of the disease. This is frequently true of young people contemplating starting a family. The other parent (*aa*) does not carry the gene for HD. Since the HD gene is dominant, it will rule whenever it appears in combination with its healthy allele. As the diagram indicates, half of the children of a union between a carrier and a noncarrier will inherit the disease.[18]

Normal Parent = *aa* ↓			← Carrier Parent = *Aa*
	A	*a*	
a	*Aa* (Affected)	*aa* (Normal)	
a	*Aa* (Affected)	*aa* (Normal)	

Figure 2.2. Inheritance pattern for dominant genetic conditions. The mutant gene is represented by 'A' because it is dominant and the normal gene by 'a' because it is recessive. From A. E. H. Emery, *Elements of Medical Genetics*, 4th ed. (Berkeley: University of California Press, 1975).

It is important to remember that this diagram is a *statistical* model. On *average*, half the children resulting from a union in which one parent carries the gene for a dominant disorder like HD will inherit the gene. But an average is obtained by sampling many cases. In a single family, such as that of Ian Miller, only one person, or perhaps two, or all or none, could inherit the gene. This is true because inheriting the gene is a matter of pure chance and there are not enough people in any one family to constitute a viable statistical model. As Dr. Chiu explained to Ian, each *individual* faces exactly even odds at birth—a fifty-fifty chance of inheriting the gene for HD.

Most people who inherit the HD gene begin to show symptoms of the disease in the third to fifth decade of life. Why the gene does not usually begin to take its toll until then remains a mystery. A few people do manifest the disorder in childhood; others do not show it until they are fifty or sixty. It sometimes happens, therefore, that three or four generations are simultaneously involved with the disease at various levels.

As an example, let us consider a family in which a sixty-year-old (*A*) is in the advanced stages of the disease. This means that *A*'s forty-year-old offspring (*B*) is at risk for the disease. Let us assume that *B* has not, as yet, shown any symptoms of the disorder. *B*, in turn, has a twenty-year-old son or daughter (*C*) who knows that the gene is in the family but is also uncertain about his or her eventual fate. Finally, *C* may be the parent of a baby (*D*) whose future depends upon what eventually happens to its grandparent and parent.

Each generation in this example is threatened by Huntington's disease but each has a different statistical relationship to it. *B* knows that he is at risk because his parent definitely has the disease. But *C* must wait until *B* either shows symptoms of the disorder or reaches an advanced age without symptoms before he (*C*) can even know whether he is at risk. The fate of baby *D* is governed by what happens to both *B* and *C*. If *B* reaches an advanced age (sixty to seventy years) without any sign of the disease, then *C* can be reasonably assured that *B* did not inherit the gene and therefore could not have passed it on. This is significant comfort for both *C* and *D*. The problem is that by the time *B* reaches the age of seventy, *C* will be fifty years old, and baby *D* will have reached the age of thirty.

If *B* does get the disease, this confirms that *C* is definitely at risk. *D* would then have to wait to see what happens to his parent to know whether he (*D*) is also at risk. Until *C* actually shows symptoms of the disease, *D* can truly be said to be at risk of being at risk. There is a danger here because, as he matures, *D* may be tempted to conclude that the disease constitutes an insignificant threat for him. From the reflection that *B* must demonstrate the disease in order to confirm that *C* is at risk and then *C* must also show signs to put him (*D*) at risk—in which case he may *still* escape the disease—*D* may rationalize that he faces very little risk at all. This is not a realistic way to approach a hereditary disorder as serious as Huntington's disease. The critical reality is that the HD gene is in the family and it carries a very high risk of recurrence. It is quite normal and healthy to hope for the best, but one should also try to be prepared for the worst.

Probably the best attitude is one poised between hope and preparedness at a point determined by an honest appraisal of the facts. This point of balance, which is difficult enough to achieve when all the facts are known and understood, cannot be achieved at all in the presence of ignorance. An incomplete understanding of HD can as easily result in undue pessimism as in unrealistic optimism. For example, some people who know that they are at risk for HD go through their entire lives believing that the risk is 50 percent. As we shall see in the next chapter, this is an intolerable burden to bear and, strictly speaking, it isn't true. The recurrence risk declines with advancing years. For a person who reaches the age of forty-two years without showing any sign of the disease, the statistical risk of recurrence is down from 50 percent to about 30 percent. There are still three chances in ten that he will get the disease, but there are seven chances in ten that he will not. At the age of fifty-five, the person has about one chance in ten of getting the disorder.[19]

Of course, it would be a mistake to confuse high statistical probability with certainty. Although it is true that 90 percent of cases become apparent before the person reaches his or her late fifties, this statistic is cold comfort if you happen to be the one who has an extremely late onset. On the other hand, it is important to keep in mind that the risk does decline slowly with each passing year. For a forty-five-year-old person who is free of symptoms to speak of being 50 percent at risk is inaccurate. By that age the risk is considerably lower.

HUNTINGTON'S DISEASE AND THE BRAIN

Exactly what is responsible for HD, and exactly what mechanisms trigger its onset, are not now known. Overt physiological and psychological changes that take place after onset of the disease, on the other hand, are known in some detail. When the causative dominant gene, which for years has remained quiescent or perhaps has been held in check by other forces within the body, begins to take its toll, brain cells (called neurons) begin to die. Unlike cells in other parts of the body, they cannot be replaced. The brain slowly deteriorates and, eventually, symptoms of Huntington's disease begin to appear. With the brain unable to fulfill its normal functions, the affected person gradually loses control over voluntary muscle movements. We can approach a clearer understanding of this and other symptoms of Huntington's disease by examining the structure and function of neurons.

Neurons come in many shapes and sizes. They may be likened to a human hand with many threadlike fingers, called dendrites, and a long, thin thumb, called the axon. A nerve signal, in the form of an electrical impulse, originates in the cell body and speeds out over the axon to communicate with other cells in the brain. The dendrite fingers provide the avenue for incoming signals. The brain works by utilizing an enormous network of neurons. Each communicates with others over points of contact called synapses, where messages are exchanged by chemicals known as neurotransmitters. One authority has estimated that the human brain has 100,000,000,000 neurons—a number roughly equal to the number of stars in our galaxy—and a typical neuron may have anywhere from 1,000 to 10,000 synapses.[20]

In effect, the neuron acts as a tiny secreting gland to either excite or inhibit action on the part of adjacent cells. When a neuron receives a message to initiate action that is stronger than the message to inhibit it, it relays a "yes" message to its neighbors, influencing their response. Put another way, tens of thousands of millions of individual neurons are functioning as tiny prototypes of the brain itself, receiving, processing, and transmitting information in order to produce an appropriate response.[21] It is a delicate and wonderful process. If the process is disturbed, perhaps as a result of injury or illness, the results can be very serious.

The progressive degeneration of neurons in certain portions of the brain causes the gradual appearance of the symptoms associated with Huntington's disease.[22] Post-mortem examination of HD brains reveals that they have an average weight of 150 to 500

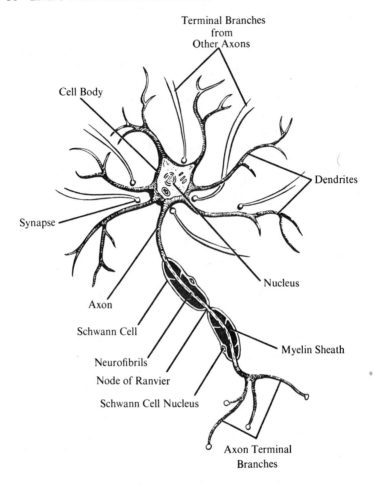

Figure 2.3. Nerve cell. This highly schematic drawing shows part of the cell body and axon cut away to reveal internal structures. From *Explorers of the Brain* by Leonard A. Stevens, illustrated by Edd Ashe. Copyright © 1971 by Leonard A. Stevens. Reprinted by permission of Alfred A. Knopf, Inc.

grams less than normal brains. They also show various biochemical abnormalities which can be measured. These abnormalities involve the balance of vital chemicals that act as neurotransmitters.[23]

In the early 1970s, Professor Thomas L. Perry of the University of British Columbia reported a marked deficiency of a neurotransmitter called gamma-aminobutyric acid (GABA) in some key regions of the brains of persons who had died with Huntington's disease.[24] Normal voluntary muscle movements, as well as normal thought and emotional reactions, depend on a proper balance in the brain of a large number of neurotransmitters, including GABA, glutamic acid, dopamine, noradrenaline, serotonin, and acetylcholine. GABA is an important inhibitory neurotransmitter—a chemical which, when it is released at synapses, acts to prevent the firing of neighboring neurons. Soon after Professor Perry's discovery, other researchers found that the enzyme which makes GABA, glutamic acid decarboxylase (GAD), had decreased activity in the same brain areas of patients dying with Huntington's disease where GABA content was low.[25]

GABA research was hailed by some as the long-awaited breakthrough in the search for the ultimate cause of HD. Great hope was held that development of a substance which imitated the action of GABA could lead to a form of drug therapy that relieved at least some of the symptoms of HD in much the same way as the drug L-DOPA had proven useful in the treatment of Parkinson's disease.[26] This optimistic expectation proved premature. As research continued, it became clear that the mystery of Huntington's disease would not be solved so easily. A GABA deficiency was certainly implicated in HD, but it was only one detail in a very complex picture.[27]

Researchers were also interested in the relationship between HD and the other neurotransmitters. For example, scientists were intrigued by the activity of the neurotransmitter dopamine, which seems to be involved in both Parkinson's disease and Huntington's disease. The biochemical findings in Parkinson's disease research helped to confirm the presumption of a fundamental metabolic defect in Huntington's disease.[28] Scientists learned that a certain class of drugs which may produce unwanted side effects resembling the symptoms of Parkinsonism can sometimes be useful in controlling the involuntary muscle movements associated with HD. It seemed possible that, whereas in Parkinsonism there is a deficiency of dopamine activity in an area of the brain called the striatum, in Huntington's disease there might be a relative overactivity of dopamine.[29]

(a)

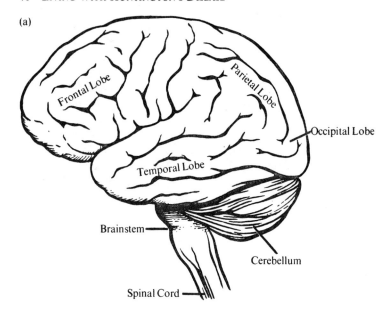

(b)

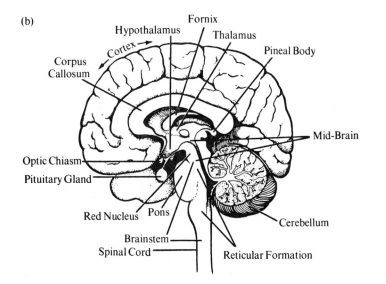

(c)   Hemispheres
                            (Right)   (Left)

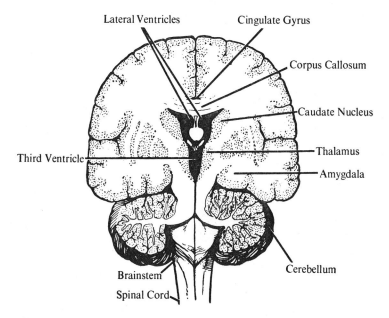

Figure 2.4. Three views of the human brain: (a) left hemisphere, showing cortex as viewed from the side; (b) vertical section cutting down between the two hemispheres and through brainstem and cerebellum; (c) both hemispheres, shown by vertical section cutting across organ to the spinal cord. From *Explorers of the Brain* by Leonard A. Stevens, illustrated by Edd Ashe. Copyright © 1971 by Leonard A. Stevens. Reprinted by permission of Alfred A. Knopf, Inc.

During the next few years, intensive research in several laboratories on autopsied brains of patients who died with Huntington's disease disclosed that at least two neurotransmitters besides GABA are sometimes deficient in the most affected brain areas. Acetylcholine is probably reduced in the brains of about half of all HD patients at death, as shown by a reduction in the activity of the enzyme that synthesizes acetylcholine.[30] There is also a deficiency of another neurotransmitter, called substance P, in at least two brain areas.[31] The increased activity of dopamine which has already been noted may simply indicate that neurons which produce dopamine, and release it as a neurotransmitter, have been spared, while many neurons that utilize GABA, acetylcholine, or substance P as their neurotransmitters are either malfunctioning or dead.[32] In any case, most scientists now believe that in the brains of persons suffering from Huntington's disease there is a serious neurotransmitter imbalance, with a relative overactivity of dopamine and a relative underactivity of GABA, acetylcholine, substance P, and possibly additional neurotransmitters.

All of the questions raised by GABA and dopamine research apply to the other neurotransmitters believed to be implicated in Huntington's disease. To what extent do neurotransmitter imbalances cause the disorder, and to what extent are they themselves caused by a more basic problem? Professor André Barbeau in Montreal has suggested that the real cause of Huntington's disease may have nothing to do with neurotransmitter metabolism. He believes that the fundamental mechanism of the disease is more likely related to abnormalities in the membranes of certain neurons.[33]

Neurotransmitter imbalances and cell membrane abnormalities are only two of many areas of active inquiry in the search for the fundamental mechanism of Huntington's disease. Could the basic problem be an inability of brain cells to grow properly? Is there a critical deficiency of some trace metal(s)? Is some malfunction of the endocrine glands (secretory glands responsible for a wide range of important regulatory actions) at fault? Is some autoimmune reaction responsible?[34]

Although definitive answers to these vital questions are still beyond our grasp, it is reassuring to know that researchers in many countries are working diligently to expand our knowledge. More progress has been made toward understanding HD in the last decade than in the whole previous history of the disease, and there is certainly reason to hope that a stroke of luck, a brilliant insight, or painstaking labor will produce a breakthrough. But optimism must be tempered with caution. As our knowledge about Huntington's disease has grown, so has our knowledge of the immensity of the challenge.

For the present, we must assume that HD may not be explained for many years. People involved with the disease must make their decisions according to what they know to be true now rather than what they hope will happen in the future. If HD is eventually explained and conquered, that will probably happen as a result of the combined contributions of many people working carefully and patiently over a long period of time. It is one of the most difficult and baffling of many hundreds of genetic conditions. We cannot expect that it will yield its secrets overnight.

3

Meeting the Challenge of Living "At Risk" for Huntington's Disease

Being at risk is dying a little each time you drop a spoon.
Being at risk is looking at your brothers and sisters,
wondering which one of you will be the first to go. This constant
pressure, day in, day out, year after year, takes a heavy toll. . . .
I feel at times that being at risk has taken away my right
to love and be loved.

People at risk for Huntington's disease must learn to live with an unrelenting challenge. Because HD is a late-onset disorder for which no predictive test is presently possible, every child of a parent who develops the disease must live with terrible uncertainty for many years waiting to find out how the genetic dice were rolled before he was born. This constant pressure can become so intense that it virtually disables some people. Persons who might otherwise lead healthy lives may become so "locked in" to their risk for Huntington's disease that, even though they may not have inherited the defective gene, the threat of the disease incapacitates them, or causes fundamental personality changes. On the other hand, many who are at risk for HD live quietly heroic lives, coping daily with the challenge in a constructive and inspirational way.

What accounts for the greatly varying success that different people have in coping with their risk for Huntington's disease? A little has been said, and more will be said in later chapters, about the vital role played by various public institutions. Central to this chapter, however, is the subject of self-help, which is surely the best point of departure in considering most human problems. What can those at risk for HD do to help *themselves?* Secondarily, what can family members and friends do to help a person who is at risk for Huntington's disease?

The best guiding principle, not surprisingly, is urged by common sense, and has general applicability in human affairs. It is, very simply, to be realistic. The most unhappy errors made by those who are subject to HD's spell of uncertainty are errors resulting from a failure to be realistic and honest about the disease. It is a failure, as we shall see, that can take either of two forms. Those concerned about a risk for HD can err in the direction of pessimism, by exaggerating the worst possibilities and ignoring the reasons for hope and encouragement; or they can err in the direction of denial and neglect, rationalizing away or deliberately ignoring the serious questions that should concern them. In this chapter, therefore, we will consider both the positive and negative ways in which people respond to the challenge of living at risk for HD, and from these examples, we will try to distill a measure of practical wisdom.

ERRORS OF PESSIMISM

Unfortunately, some people give up before the struggle even begins. They treat the fifty-fifty risk factor as if it meant 100 percent certainty that they will get the disease. This feeling is inevitable from time to time. No one can maintain a constant, evenly balanced attitude toward the disease. But any wholly negative feeling should not be allowed to become a dominant force in life. It is quite useless for people living at risk for Huntington's disease to sink into permanent despair, lamenting their fate as if God had cursed them. No good purpose is served—and many potentially happy days are wasted—by exaggerating both the odds of getting the disease and the dreadfulness of the disease itself.

It is safe to say that everyone wavers often between positive and negative attitudes. But it is particularly important for the person who is at risk for Huntington's disease to keep the occasional depression and negative impulse within bounds. Positive yet honest attitudes are not simply desirable, but essential, and should be deliberately cultivated.

People who assume not only that they will get the disease but that when they do it will take the worst possible form could be said to suffer from the "worst-case syndrome." They fear that they will become "vegetables," and they erroneously view the disease as fatal or totally disabling, virtually from the moment of diagnosis. This is an extreme error of pessimism. It is worth remembering that, even if the disease does appear, life is not over. As Marjorie Guthrie has commented, "I hate it when Huntington's is described as a fatal disease. Fatal implies that your life is over tomorrow. Life itself is a fatal disease and being born is the first symptom."[1]

One of the most disturbing aspects of Huntington's disease is the prospect of failing mental capacity. People feel that they can live with involuntary muscle movement, but not without their minds. This is what they mean when they speak of becoming a "vegetable" or turning into a "cabbage." What inelegant and inaccurate language we use! A person who suffers from even the most serious mental or physical illness is *not* a "vegetable" and should never be referred to in that way. I suspect that if we were held publicly accountable for comments like this we would be more accurate and considerate in our choice of words.

The fear of mental and physical deterioration is often linked with a fear of prolonged dependency. Young people who are not married worry that the threat of the disease, and the dependency it could cause, might prevent anyone from loving them or sharing their life on a permanent basis. Married people fear not only their own fate but what the disease could mean for their spouses and families. A few even declare that they would rather commit suicide than be a burden to themselves, their relatives, or society.

It is perhaps not surprising that many who make the worst-case assumption, identifying their future with a picture of Huntington's disease at its worst, contemplate suicide. One study of thirty-five persons at risk for HD found that "approximately half the sample felt they would seriously consider suicide as an option if and when they *started* to deteriorate" (emphasis added). Everyone who participated in the study was "painfully aware that the disease is terminal, but for them the termination comes not at the moment of death but at the moment of diagnosis. Most fantasize the period following diagnosis to be a prolonged and unproductive wait on death row."[2]

There is no doubt that many people act on these feelings. The suicide rate among HD patients is estimated at seven times the American average.[3] But the mistaken perception that life ends at the moment of positive diagnosis is tragic even when it does not lead to suicide. It simply ignores the years of productive and self-reliant living that are almost always possible after the onset of symptoms of Huntington's disease.

This is not to suggest, of course, that persons at risk for HD have no reason to be concerned about the future. The disease is serious, and living at risk for it is an unusual and extraordinarily demanding life situation. None of us likes to contemplate the prospect of physical and mental deterioration—even if we all face exactly that in the normal process of aging—and when we are forced to think about it because we are known to be at high risk of inheriting an incurable disease, then life can become very difficult indeed. Under these circumstances, it is understandable that some people develop self-destructive attitudes. But these people are often unfair to themselves and to those around them.

Probably the most persistent result of excessive pessimism is a preoccupation with the disease. Persons at risk for HD become "disease-wise and doctor-shy."[4] Far from denying the disease, they become vigilant symptom-watchers, continually on the alert for any subtle sign of HD's onset. Sometimes relatives and friends make matters worse by joining the vigil. Every slip or stumble, muscular tic, dropped spoon, forgotten telephone number, or bout of depression is misinterpreted as an early indicator of the presence of the disease. The person at risk watches himself, and is watched by other members of the family, as if he were an experimental animal. Consequently, although getting HD is somewhat less than a fifty-fifty possibility, constant vigilance makes many people "one-hundred percent miserable worrying while they are healthy."[5]

Those at risk for Huntington's disease should strive to separate realistic concern over the illness from unrelated problems. It is often tempting to make HD more troublesome than it already is. Dr. Nancy Wexler, a clinical psychologist and Executive Director of the United States Commission for the Control of Huntington's Disease and Its Consequences, has written, "The prospect of having Huntington's disease can feed into every conflict, and each problem can be interpreted in terms of Huntington's disease. . . . For some it may be easier to lay the blame with Huntington's disease rather than face vulnerabilities, failures, or weaknesses which have nothing to do with the disease."[6]

There is a fine line between being aware of the disease and becoming preoccupied by it, a line that is sometimes crossed unknowingly and with unhappy results. For example, a man in Canada recalled exploding in anger when his wife mentioned her concern over nervous movements in her hands. He later realized that he had been watching her for signs of the disease. In his anxious wish that she should escape the disorder, he subconsciously blamed her for openly suggesting that she might be showing symptoms. As it turned out, she did not have the disease. But her doubts and distress while there was still uncertainty were needlessly compounded by her husband's unsympathetic response to her attempt to discuss the matter with him.

In a similar case in England, a woman constantly watched her husband for early signs of the disease. She could not resist commenting on every little "abnormality," imagined or otherwise. She needlessly focused attention on minor quirks which would have gone entirely unnoticed in anyone not known to be at risk for HD. The threat of the disease was kept in the foreground at all times, greatly increasing the burden of concern borne by her husband. Her unconstructive behavior did not arise from conscious cruelty. On the contrary, she was well-intentioned. She loved her husband and saw herself as trying to help. Her counterproductive actions had their impulse, rather, in repressed anxiety and frustration over her powerlessness.

Symptom-watching can become so exaggerated that persons at risk for HD feel deprived of the opportunity to lead a normal life. One man remarked to Dr. Wexler that he envied his wife's "right to be clumsy."[7] A twenty-three-year-old woman complained that she felt she had no right to be herself or participate in some normal activities: "I get messages like: You have no right to your feelings. You can't feel angry. If you feel scared you'd better hide it. Don't even cry." It is little wonder that many who are at risk prefer to keep it a secret. No one wants to be a center of morbid or over-solicitous attention.

Although most people experience a series of changing attitudes in their continuing process of adjustment, that process should not be overshadowed by gloomy or excessively pessimistic notions. A 50 percent risk is not 100 percent certainty. And getting the disease is not the end of the world. One man who eventually got the disease recalled several years of "depression, withdrawal, quietness, secretiveness and ruminating about whether all the struggles were worthwhile." He overcame these obstacles and plunged into a program of community action to combat HD, working as best he could to help alleviate the plight of others who had the disorder. This activity continued at a lively pace for more than a decade after he was diagnosed with the disease.[8]

ERRORS OF DENIAL AND NEGLECT

Some people who are at risk for Huntington's disease attempt to cope with the problem by pretending that it does not exist. They ignore it and deny that it could possibly affect them. They do not talk about HD, nor do they seriously consider it when they contemplate having a family. The threat of the disease may be carelessly dismissed with the flick of a wrist and a casual comment like, "When your number is up, your number is up." This nonchalant attitude may be comforting to some people, but it is neither a responsible nor a constructive reaction to the possible presence of the disease. The defective gene, unfortunately, is not influenced by an attitude of denial. Huntington's disease will not go away simply because people wish that it would. A parent who carries the defective gene, but who ignores the disorder or represses discussion of its possible consequences, will still transmit the risk to the next generation. Unbelievable suffering is perpetuated by people who mistakenly think that the best way to deal with Huntington's disease is to ignore it.

An attitude of denial is very tempting, because people who are at risk for HD often feel that they are living with a genetic time bomb that could explode at any moment. This is especially true for those who, during childhood, witnessed the gradual deterioration of an affected parent. These people may either exaggerate the threat of the disease or attempt to deny it entirely. An observed pattern of vigorous self-deception among persons with this unfortunate childhood experience led Dr. Wexler to conclude that "the nature of the children's early exposure to Huntington's disease appeared to be critical in determining their adult adjustment to their own genetic risk."[9]

The horrific impressions created by childhood exposure to parents afflicted with HD may be indelible, but these impressions should not be allowed to prey on an adult's better judgment. For one thing, such memories, if they go back even a few years, misrepresent the facts about HD today. While still far from ideal, the treatment and care of HD patients has improved so markedly in the last decade that it bears little resemblance to the unimaginative and callous way many patients have been treated in the past. Although some patients are still badly mistreated—a cause for serious concern—it is wrong for individuals at risk to assume, for example, that they will end up in an insane asylum.

Persons at risk for HD sometimes view the disorder in "the context of crime and punishment" or guilt.[10] They may see the disease as a punishment for their sins, or even for sins committed in the distant past by their ancestors. Perhaps the Christian belief that the sin of Adam was visited on all future generations has something to do with this notion. Whatever its source, the belief that HD, or any hereditary disease, represents a judgment or family curse is absurd. Huntington's disease is a biochemical phenomenon whose transmission is regulated by genetic law. It has nothing to do with vice or virtue, sin or sanctity, crime or punishment.

Sadly, some people who are not themselves at risk for HD unwittingly contribute to the belief that the disease is a product of crime or misbehavior. Dr. Wexler tells of a police matron who threatened a twelve-year-old girl by telling her that she had better behave or she would get the same disease that afflicted her mother.

One consequence of the crime and punishment view is a natural hope of escaping the disease through "bargaining." The police matron encouraged the twelve-year-old girl to bargain good behavior for possible escape from the disease. Many adults bargain, in effect, by assuming that they can guarantee their good health by paying some price. Dr. Wexler interviewed one woman who vowed that, if spared, she would be "a good Samaritan and care for the rest." Others believed that they could bargain with God by praying and doing good deeds. Still others felt safe simply because they had "always been lucky."

Bargaining helps to water the garden of myth and misconception which seems to flourish whenever an incurable disease is involved. People manage to persuade themselves that they will escape (or not escape, as the case may be) because the disease only strikes the firstborn, or the youngest, or the second male or third female. Sometimes the exchange offered in a bargain is worked out in peculiar detail. One woman was absolutely convinced that she would escape the disease if she visited the hospital bed of her affected mother twice weekly. A man swore that regular baths in an isolated natural spring would guarantee him immunity. A fundamentalist preacher convinced several families that giving large sums of money to his church would deliver them from the disease. There are enough myths, legends, and swindles about immunity from HD to fill several volumes. The simple truth is that HD follows well-known genetic laws, and no amount of bargaining—no matter how hopeful or well-intentioned—will change those laws. Bargaining doesn't work.

People bargain because it is difficult to accept a random calamity without seeking a rational explanation. All of us are reluctant to admit that any disaster is truly random, because that very admission makes us more painfully aware of our personal vulnerability. It is commonly said, for example, that someone who is mugged should never have been on the street alone at that hour in the first place; or that a whole city wiped out by a cyclone or tornado was itself to blame for not heeding warnings or taking adequate precautions in advance. These arguments help us to "explain" the event, and to reassure us that we can avoid a similar fate.

Dr. Wexler has observed that most people who are at risk for HD, consciously or subconsciously, believe that its apparent genetic randomness is somehow mediated by a moral universe. This perspective has something in common with bargaining, but it may serve a useful purpose. For example, many people seek a religious explanation or solution. They reason that if God "should choose to inflict the disease, then it is not randomly assigned but made meaningful through God's will."[11] They may believe that they can influence God to intervene on their behalf, or they may simply find great comfort and hope in religious faith.

For some people, these two aspects of religious conviction overlap. They try to influence God through prayer, and they draw strength from their religious faith whether or not prayer is an effective weapon against the disease. Other people with deep religious beliefs feel that it is inappropriate to petition God to intervene directly. Their prayers are intended to ease their adjustment to whatever happens, or are offered on behalf of others. Individual views vary greatly, but there is no doubt that for many people prayer and religious faith are constructive ways to respond to the presence of Huntington's disease in their lives.

Any attitude toward HD which fails to acknowledge and realistically deal with the facts about the disease can have unhappy results, not only for the person at risk but for friends and family. Honest acknowledgment of the facts is essential for everyone's well-being. Many couples have had quite successful and joyous marriages in full awareness that one partner is at risk for Huntington's disease. Even when the disease appears, these couples make the necessary adjustments and continue to find meaning in life with each other. Generally speaking, the people who cope best are those who have learned about HD at an early age and who discuss it freely and openly. Tragedy is much more likely to strike when the facts about HD are concealed or ignored.[12]

Being informed and keeping others informed about Huntington's disease is important, but the disorder is not an easy thing to discuss, even at the best of times. Young people often have trouble talking about it. If you are getting serious about someone and thinking about a permanent relationship, how and when do you introduce the subject of Huntington's disease? Isn't the whole thing so difficult and so terrible that the less said about it the better? No. Even in such a painful situation it is better to be open. The worst possible results of being honest are not as bad as the likely consequences of secretiveness. Although Huntington's disease is not a subject you would chat about on the first date, there usually comes a time in an ongoing relationship when a person can simply say, "There is something very important I want you to know. Potentially it affects us both, and I want to talk to you about it." With that start, it is less difficult to present the essential facts about HD. Then the person who has just been informed about the disease can be given plenty of time to reflect on it and react as he or she sees fit. If the relationship ends as a result of this conversation, far better that it should end here than after permanent commitments have been made. But the person at risk should not feel that the relationship *will* necessarily end here.

Informing children is also difficult. Fearing that exposure to the disease may destroy the self-esteem of a child who is at risk, well-meaning parents may seek to isolate the child from the disease and from anyone who has the disorder. As a general rule, it is better for both the child and the parent to deal with the presence of the disease more directly and honestly. If a parent is affected by the disease, a child may begin to ask questions at an early age. Information about the disease should be given as the child asks and shows an ability to understand what is being explained. If the parent is at risk but has no symptoms of the disease, the child will probably never have occasion to ask questions about it. Parents may then be tempted to defer discussing the disorder on the grounds that they may escape it. They may reason that if they do escape, there is no cause to worry the children, and if they don't escape, there is still plenty of time to explain the problem.

The obvious fallacy in this reasoning is that a parent who begins to show symptoms at the age of forty or forty-five may have a child of twenty or twenty-five who has already made major life commitments. What happens then? Withholding information which has a direct bearing on some of life's most crucial decisions is not a favor to anyone. Children have a right to be informed about any real or potential genetic risk in their future. Parents who fail to inform their children may be using the alleged welfare of the children as a convenient excuse for not dealing with an unpleasant and difficult problem.

Children who are introduced gradually but early to the reality of the disease are almost always better able to manage their own risk later in life than those who are kept in ignorance for years and then have the facts dropped upon them like a bomb. When they are informed relatively late in life, they may feel that they have been betrayed, and their lives may be hurt in tangible ways.

This very thing happened to a young woman in Queensland, Australia. She had been married for six years before she learned that her father had Huntington's disease. Her parents, who had known all along that the gene was in the family, attempted to "let her lead a normal life for as long as possible" by keeping the facts from her. They naturally hoped that her father would be lucky and escape the disease, leaving her and her children free from risk. When the young woman learned that her father had the disease, she promptly told her husband. He responded badly. He cursed and said, "I certainly didn't buy into this when we got married." Then he packed up and left her to provide alone for their two small children. In a misguided attempt to help their daughter lead a normal life, these parents concealed information from her which she desperately needed before she got married. Concealment only delayed the day when she had to face the problem. It also made that experience much more complicated and traumatic than it should have been.

Finally, getting Huntington's disease should not mean that a parent must also face the prospect of separation from his or her children. Nor should children be "protected" from the disease against their will by being isolated from an affected parent. Self-deception can develop into just as serious a problem for the person at risk who has never seen the disease as it can for someone who witnessed the disorder in an affected relative.

CONCLUSION: A POSITIVE APPROACH

Researchers have discovered that various stages of adjustment are common among people who must cope with any degenerative illness. Dr. Elisabeth Kübler-Ross has noted, for example, that these stages usually involve a transition from denial and isolation to anger, bargaining, depression, and finally acceptance and hope.[13] In the case of HD and other neurological diseases, the usual stages of adjustment may be affected by biochemical changes which are part of the disease process. Anger and emotional outbursts may be linked to disease-related changes in the patient's brain, not to more easily managed psychological causes.

Nevertheless, it is clear that most people who must cope with either the possibility or the presence of Huntington's disease go through a series of adjustments, which may involve denial, anger, bargaining, depression, etc. To the extent that such unconstructive responses are necessary for the transition to a healthy adjustment, it is perhaps unfair to stop at calling them undesirable. But it is important to prevent negative feelings from dominating permanently. A determinedly positive attitude, tempered by a realistic assessment of the facts, constitutes a mature and constructive approach to the challenge of living at risk for Huntington's disease.

Positive factors can be emphasized without distorting the reality of the situation. For one thing, it should be remembered that the risk for Huntington's disease declines with age; not all cases are totally incapacitating; some people are in their seventies and get along quite well even though they have the disease; many live productive lives for years after the disease has been diagnosed; new drugs and new methods of treatment mean a brighter future for HD patients, and unprecedented research activity promises new hope for the future.[14] When the condition of actually having Huntington's disease is seen as less threatening, then the anxiety over being at risk is reduced.

A positive attitude is easier to cultivate when you remember that you are not alone. There are others in this world who face similar or more difficult challenges. Moreover, persons who are at risk for HD and who assume that no one will love them or willingly stand by them are often doing an injustice to others. Many husbands, wives, parents, children, brothers, sisters, other relatives, and friends are intimately committed to the struggle against HD. They are wholeheartedly involved in trying to improve the quality of life for those who face the disease. They do not view the prospect of living with someone who has HD as an intolerable burden. Of course the possibility that the person living at risk could inherit a serious disease that has implications for other members of the family cannot be ignored, but otherwise life goes on.

The support of family and friends cannot be very effective if the person who is at risk isolates himself from others. One of the simplest and most effective mechanisms for coping with HD at any level is to talk about it. You may confide in your spouse, another relative, a friend, or perhaps your clergyman or doctor. Whoever you turn to, it is important to be able to discuss your worries and problems in a comfortable atmosphere without fear or embarrassment. Too often, a "conspiracy of silence" envelops the disease.[15] Even married couples sometimes avoid the subject, either because they are afraid of it or because neither wishes to draw the other's attention to it. While it may not be a topic you want to raise every night at the dinner table, neither should it become a taboo which is never mentioned at all.

With this in mind, a few words are in order for friends and family of those at risk for HD. When Huntington's disease is discussed, those who are *not* at risk should guard against coping with their own anxieties by placing additional burdens on the person who is at risk. This tendency, as we have seen, can easily steal over even the well-intentioned as a result of subconscious frustration. But it can arise from a number of causes and take a variety of forms. When a thirty-five-year-old woman in Montreal took leave from work to care for her affected mother, her "friends" beat a track to her door to pour out their own troubles —failing marriages, delinquent children, obesity, etc. They offered no practical assistance and used the woman as an outlet for their own problems, presumably because they were satisfied that they were doing her a favor merely by being there. She absorbed it all with a smile and helpful advice. But not everyone can carry heavy personal loads and also help those who are only lightly burdened. Persons at risk for HD have enough to do without shouldering the psychological problems of others. One of the best things other members of the family can do is learn to listen. It is a skill which few people possess.

People who are trying to help should give careful thought when they offer advice. They may mean well when they encourage a friend not to worry because "life is full of risks—you could step into the street and get run over by a bus at any time," but this is not a helpful observation. The feeling of anxiety over the possible future onset of Huntington's disease is not mitigated by thinking about irrelevant alternative misfortunes. In any event, who wants to be run over by a bus?

The worst fear of people who are at risk for Huntington's disease is that they will eventually get the disease and life will become meaningless for them. For most people, death itself is not nearly as fearful as the possibility of years of meaningless suffering. It is appropriate, therefore, to conclude this chapter with some brief observations about meaning in life.

Persons at risk for HD share a view common to most people when they think in terms of what they "expect from life" or what they "hope to get out of life." When they imagine a situation in which their ability to "get something out of life" is reduced, they naturally doubt whether life, in such a case, would be worth living.

It may be useful to consider meaning in life from an alternative viewpoint. The meaning of life is not, after all, the same for everybody. It varies from person to person according to a multitude of circumstances. And for each person it varies from day to day, even from hour to hour. The meaning of life constantly changes, but *never ceases to exist*. It exists even in suffering. Often it exists especially in suffering. That is fortunate, because suffering is an inevitable part of life. Granted, some will suffer more than others; but meeting that reality bravely imparts a potent meaning to life for as long as it lasts.[16]

Meaning in life does not depend on luck or any special happenstance. It is not a product of whether or not we get rich, become famous, or acquire power. It is not even the result of whether or not we get Huntington's disease. Meaning in life is actualized by the way we respond to the questions and challenges life brings to each of us. By responding well, we infuse life with significance. Therefore, a conscious effort to cope constructively with Huntington's disease can lead to cumulative victories. By seizing the initiative and not giving up, we can draw strength from dealing effectively with each new day. Every challenge well met adds to the proof that this business of living at risk for Huntington's disease *is* manageable. The confidence grows that even should the disease appear, it can be met with courage and energy.

4

Genetic Counseling

I have become acutely aware of how little I know about Huntington's disease, both as a person and as a physician.

After Mother's HD diagnosis, she and Daddy had consulted the parish priest about a birth control dispensation because of the hereditary factor. The priest said there were no exceptions.

Genetic counseling is a widely used but loosely defined term. Many medical dictionaries omit it entirely. Those that attempt a definition may offer nothing more specific than "advice based on genetic or partly genetic information." This failure to define the term precisely becomes more understandable when we note that it was not coined until 1947, when Sheldon Reed of the Dight Institute of Human Genetics in Minneapolis used it in a contemporary sense. At that time there were only a handful of genetic counseling centers in the United States. Now there are many hundreds throughout the world.[1]

In 1974 an ad hoc committee sponsored by Canada's National Genetics Foundation published a detailed definition which soon gained wide acceptance:

> Genetic counseling is a communication process which deals with the human problems associated with the occurrence, or risk of occurrence, of a genetic disorder in a family. This process involves an attempt by one or more appropriately trained persons to help the individual or family to (1) comprehend the medical facts, including the diagnosis, probable course of the

disorder, and the available management; (2) appreciate the way heredity contributes to the disorder, and the risk of recurrence in specified relatives; (3) understand the alternatives for dealing with the risk of recurrence; (4) choose the course of action which seems to them appropriate in view of their risk, their ethical and religious standards, and to act in accordance with that decision; and (5) to make the best possible adjustment to the disorder in an affected family member and/or the risk of recurrence of that disorder.[2]

This definition describes an ideal situation. Its emphasis is properly on effective communication by trained persons who are able to offer accurate information and sustained support.[3] Unfortunately, this is not always possible. Most people with serious genetic disorders will never see a formally trained genetic counselor. Many must rely on the trusted family physician; and even the most conscientious of general practitioners find it impossible to keep up with the flood of material now appearing in the field of human genetics. More than a thousand single-gene defects have been identified in man.[4] To complicate matters, a family physician may have practiced for years without encountering a single case of an autosomal, dominant genetic disorder like Huntington's disease. Not only does misdiagnosis become a grave danger, but initial counseling may be based on assumptions and values which have little or nothing to do with empirical risk factors, inheritance patterns, and the special problems that are usually associated with degenerative neurological disorders. The potential value of the general practitioner in this area of medicine is enormous, but anyone who is well acquainted with Huntington's disease can cite examples of grievously misguided advice, or no advice at all, that was given by a medically trained person who should have known better.[5]

Some people have been told that only boys can inherit the disease. Others have been told that only girls inherit it. Some are told that if you don't have it by age thirty-five you will never get it. All this "advice" is incorrect. The family physician of a New York woman at risk for Huntington's disease told her to ignore her risk and have as many children as she wished. He said, "Life is a risk for us all. The fate of each of us is in the hands of God."[6] This philosophy may or may not be true, but it has more to do with theology than with the science of genetics. The doctor failed to help his patient comprehend her own risk. He did not inform her of the recurrence risk for her children. He told her nothing about the potential burden of the disease. His advice was inadequate, irresponsible, and potentially highly destructive.

Effective genetic counseling depends on accurate and informed communication, but it depends also on a genuinely positive attitude. There is a growing appreciation that counseling is a potent therapeutic tool where incurable degenerative disorders like HD are concerned.[7] Some general practitioners offer sound advice, but overshadow it with a note of hopelessness. At a time when the counselee most needs strong and positive support, all he or she gets is a message of resignation and despair. It may also happen that the facts about HD are unloaded like a bombshell on an unsuspecting person, and no arrangement is made for further counseling or follow-up. It is not surprising that when genetic counseling is conducted in such haphazard and insensitive ways it makes matters worse.

The problem is magnified when amateurs give genetic advice. This can occur quite naturally. The first genetic counseling an individual receives may come from a close relative. Among families in which the HD gene is present, one of the parents will probably be the first to inform the children about the nature of the disorder and the risk of recurrence. Some parents are well equipped to handle this task. Others are not. The possibility of misinformation being passed from one generation to the next is obvious.

The history of Huntington's disease is tragically littered with myths and misunderstandings that have been perpetuated in this way. The severe symptoms of the disease, the high recurrence risk, the inability to identify carriers or provide a cure—all of these harsh realities make rationalization and invention tempting. Every genetic counselor knows that this can lead to some bizarre myths.

Good genetic counseling can combat myth and misinformation, and it can go a long way toward helping patients and their families cope with Huntington's disease. But it is no cure.

Marjorie Guthrie has stated that, where HD is concerned, good genetic counseling helps people "live with reality—not die with it."[8] Counselors should resist the temptation to appear all-knowing or all-powerful. There is a delicate line between offering affirmative support and being overly optimistic or indulgent. Ultimately, it is the counselee who makes the decisions and lives with the reality of the disease. All the counselor can do is try to help.

EFFECTIVE COMMUNICATION

The most important element in good genetic counseling is accurate and effective communication. A person who fears that he may have a genetic disease, or be at risk of transmitting such a disease, must be able to rely on an accurate diagnosis, a precise description of the nature and consequences of the disorder, a clear explanation of recurrence risks, and a detailed analysis of alternative courses of action.

These fundamental requirements are far more complex than they might at first appear. The counselor must be aware that he is not only sharing information but is also "engaged in a complex psychodynamic process that involves the lessening of denial, the relief of guilt, the lifting of depression, the articulation of anger and, gradually, rational planning for the future."[9]

Denial, for example, is remarkably tenacious in cases of chronic, degenerative disease of late and subtle onset. The already difficult task of diagnosis may be made even more formidable by uncooperative patients or relatives who do not want to confront the possibility that a disorder like HD may be in the family. Even when given indisputable evidence that HD is present, some people will continue to act as if merely denying it will somehow make it go away. They may intentionally or inadvertently mislead a doctor or counselor. They may withhold important information. Occasionally, individuals or families may insist on their right *not* to know. Or they may try to deny the threat of the disorder by assuming that the counselor or doctor has made an error. Sometimes they may even become hostile toward the doctor for diagnosing something so serious. Doctors and counselors should be aware that such reactions are common, and should be prepared to meet them with patience and delicacy.

Imprecision in the use of important terms is another frequent barrier to effective communication. It is important in counseling to use words like genetic, congenital, hereditary, and familial with care. To employ these words as interchangeable synonyms is to invite confusion.

Since we are talking about *genetic* counseling, we should understand that *genetic disorder* refers to "an abnormality in a single gene or by an excess, deficiency, or rearrangement of the chromosomes, which may involve large numbers of genes."[10] *Congenital*, on the other hand, merely means that a given trait is present at birth. A condition (such as rubella embryopathy) may be congenital but not genetic. Huntington's disease is genetic and congenital, though not detectable at birth. A *familial* disease is a disease that "runs in families." It may be either genetic or caused by some environmental agent (such as pinworms). Victor Mc-Kusick and Robert Claiborne, in *Medical Genetics*, define *hereditary* as a synonym for *genetic*, but "in the older literature it is often used to refer to disease that appeared in parent and child through successive generations, or what we now call dominant inheritance."[11]

The counselor should always be alert to the possibility that a counselee does not comprehend, or perhaps misunderstands, the terms being used. Most people are not eager to confess their ignorance. A person may nod when a term like "autosomal dominant" is used, but may reveal incomplete understanding when asked to explain it himself. It is a good practice for the counselor to tactfully require substantive responses from the counselee to verify that key terms are clearly understood. In so far as possible, technical jargon should be avoided.

It is also enormously important that the counselor be aware of his own limitations. This is particularly true if the counselor happens to be a general practitioner who is working toward a definitive diagnosis of Huntington's disease. Misdiagnosis still occurs with distressing frequency. The consequences of misdiagnosis can be catastrophic. Diagnostic confirmation by a properly trained and equipped medical genetics unit is essential when HD or any dominant genetic disorder is involved. In these cases a diagnosis is not being made for a single individual. The whole family is automatically implicated. There must be no mistake.

Given the inherent difficulties in diagnosing a disorder like Huntington's disease, an accurate family history is an indispensable diagnostic prerequisite. The family history (or pedigree) should extend at least as far as parents, grandparents, uncles, aunts, and first cousins. Since new Huntington's disease mutations are extremely rare, a diagnosis of HD without a family pedigree indicating the presence of the gene in at least one or two previous generations would require unmistakable symptomatic evidence. Choreic movements in a patient are insufficient evidence for a diagnosis of Huntington's disease. There are at least fifty conditions which can produce involuntary muscle movement.[12]

Obtaining a family pedigree provides the counselor with an opportunity to establish a solid relationship with the counselee before entering more advanced stages of the counseling process. During this time it is important to evaluate the counselee's state of mind. Does he believe he has the disease? Does he know that he is at risk? How is he adjusting as he learns about the disorder? Are there other problems in his life which complicate the adjustment process?[13]

Persons confronted with serious, high-risk genetic disorders are naturally more likely to require extensive attention than those at low risk for relatively minor problems. Among the thousands of genetic conditions that have been identified, Huntington's disease must be accounted one of the gravest. Many other autosomal dominant defects pale by comparison. Polydactylism (too many fingers or toes), for example, is a condition which can usually be treated shortly after birth by the surgical removal of the extra digit.[14]

There are other very serious dominantly inherited diseases, but Huntington's disease is a prominent example because it has a combination of particularly insidious characteristics. Its diverse symptoms, late and subtle onset, progressive deterioration, and incurability combine to make it one of the most difficult cases that any genetic counselor will face. If counselors sometimes feel inadequate to deal with the disease, they may usefully reflect on how it must appear to those who are at risk for it or have been diagnosed with it.

People adjust to the threat of Huntington's disease in vastly different ways. Many who know that they are at risk for HD continue to live normal lives without serious internal or external conflict. Others may become depressed, even suicidal. The task for the genetic counselor is to determine who is in trouble and who is not. This is not always obvious, even after extended contact. All of us have our good days and our bad days. But there is a difference for people who are at risk for Huntington's disease. They have more reason than most to have an occasional bad day and more reason than most to be concerned about it. They must not allow a depressing day to be blown out of proportion and taken as a subtle indication of the onset of the disease. For their part, counselors face a twin challenge. They must not allow the counseling session itself to become a terribly bad day and they must help the counselee keep his or her dispirited days in proper perspective.

Reassurance, therefore, is essential, but it must not become false optimism. While well intended, too much reassurance can play into the individual's "developing set of psychological defense mechanisms including denial, rationalization, projection, and the like."[15] For example, it is perfectly accurate to say that "scientists are working on the problem," or "you have just as good a chance of escaping HD as of getting it," but constant emphasis on these themes may encourage some people to act as if the disease does not exist for them. They may ignore both the risk of recurrence and the potential burden of the disease.

David C. Wallace of Royal Newcastle Hospital in Australia has warned against the danger of turning positive support into a form of misrepresentation:

> Many patients with the disease manage to go through its progress, from the first uneasy signs of its presence to the final degeneration perhaps fifteen years later, without developing any of the more florid problems associated with it. They never require institutional treatment nor even very much in the way of psychiatric or social help. On the other hand, the disease in

some families and some individuals can be quite devastating socially, mentally, morally and physically. To gloss over these aspects of the disease as is quite often done in genetic counseling and in symposia which include lay people and supporters of the Huntington's disease associations is, I think, wrong.[16]

Despite the rapid growth of genetic counseling in the last quarter century, we still know relatively little about the psychodynamics at work during a counseling session. The more we learn, the more we are likely to realize that a multitude of factors play an important part in the counseling process. Not all of these are predictable or easily controlled. From what we already know, it is clear that there are some substantial barriers to effective communication, even in the most favorable counseling situations.

One study conducted by a team of doctors at Johns Hopkins University raises some serious questions about the effectiveness of genetic counseling. What the counselor *intends* to communicate and what is *actually* communicated may be two quite different things. In their survey of seventy-six families with various genetic disorders, the Johns Hopkins team discovered that only one-half retained a good grasp of the information given in counseling sessions that were designed to help them make decisions about having children. One-fourth retained some information, but misunderstood it; and one-fourth learned little or nothing from counseling. Statements by members of the families suggested that their attitudes were determined more by their sense of burden imposed by the disease than their awareness of precise figures for the risk of recurrence: "Although these parents knew that there were high or low risks, reproductive decisions were frequently based on factors other than risk, and . . . knowledge of specific genetic details was of importance to relatively few parents."[17]

The implications of this conclusion are far-reaching. If it is true that those at risk for HD are likely to base their reproductive decisions on the perceived burden of the disease rather than on the known risk, the counselor may wish to devote considerable time to a detailed, balanced review of the clinical facts about the disorder, rather than assuming that these facts are understood.

Doctors sometimes assume that, once the facts are explained, all reasonable couples faced with a risk for HD will decide against having children, because the disease is so serious and the risk for it so high. Certainly, Huntington's disease ranks near the top of the scale among "high risk and high burden" genetic disorders.[18] Even so, many reasonable couples do have children. This is true not only because there are rational arguments to support the case for procreation even among couples at risk for Huntington's disease, but also because sometimes a pregnancy happens without planning and a couple decides against abortion.

No genetic counselor who is attempting to communicate the harsh realities of a disorder like Huntington's disease should expect to be greeted like Santa Claus. Most of us do not welcome the bearer of bad tidings. The counseling relationship becomes even more difficult if the counselor has an aloof personality and "maintains an Olympian detachment, concerned only with the statistical probability and not the unique combination of factors entering into a counselee's personal situation. Some counselors seem to have a natural flair for establishing empathy with the counselee, but others do not."[19]

The counselor should also be aware that he can easily make a stressful situation much worse by intermingling his own coping process with that of the counselee.[20] Patients will not be reassured by counseling from someone who is having adjustment problems of his own. Nor can he counsel everyone with equal ease and success. When a significant personality conflict develops, the counselor might be well advised to guide his patient to someone else. A good counselor will not allow his ego, personal pride, or professional reputation to come before the interests and welfare of the counselee.

DIRECTIVE VS. NONDIRECTIVE COUNSELING

How prescriptive should genetic counseling be for persons who have (or could have) high risk hereditary disorders like Huntington's disease? How far is the counselor entitled to go with his advice? Should he remain strictly neutral (nondirective), or should he feel free to take a more decisive stand and direct a counselee toward what he (the counselor) believes to be the wise decision? These are questions over which genetic counselors are themselves deeply divided.[21]

The conflict between directive and nondirective counseling is most clearly drawn when couples at risk of transmitting a genetic disorder seek advice about having children. Counselors who advocate the nondirective philosophy believe that "counseling should stop at the point where an estimate of risk is given ... parents should make up their own minds what to do, without benefit (or otherwise) of further advice from the counselor."[22] Those who favor a more directive approach argue that the counselor has a responsibility to the counselee and to future generations to be more guidance-oriented, especially when disorders as serious as Huntington's disease are involved.[23] Let us examine in some detail the arguments on both sides of this important question.

The Nondirective Argument

Those who defend the nondirective approach to genetic counseling believe that the counselor has a responsibility to refrain from any attempt to influence the counselee's decisions. This is essential, they argue, for both ethical and practical reasons. Directive counseling is, in a large sense, inappropriate in a democratic society where everyone is presumed to have a sacred right to determine his own destiny. Dr. Aubrey Milunsky of the Eunice Kennedy Shriver Center in Massachusetts has noted the importance of establishing fundamental standards for genetic counseling. To open the door to directive counseling, he says, invites the counselor to visit his own religious, racial, or other convictions upon the counselee. Once the fundamental principle of neutrality is breached, abuse too easily follows. This can happen in more than one way. Sometimes the counselor is actually encouraged to be directive by a counselee, who may be asking for advice on whether or not to have children as a means of getting around making the decision himself.[24]

Advocates of nondirective counseling argue that the counselor is obligated to provide accurate information in a sympathetic but completely neutral manner. The goal is "the complete mobilization of the *positive* forces within the patient, his family, and society, for the alleviation of the particular problem."[25] Making decisions for someone else is not a positive contribution.

The counselor must be aware that he is cast in a position of considerable potential influence. As the counselee's primary source of vital information and reassurance, he may be elevated to an almost godlike position as the sole custodian of knowledge. In an age when the public has been conditioned to believe that science can work miracles, the counselor may be viewed as one who is privy to some secret answer.

When it becomes apparent that there are, as yet, no magic solutions to the most vexing problems associated with Huntington's disease, the counselee may hold his counselor personally responsible for the lack of knowledge. The counselor must be prepared for that response while at the same time exercising constant control over the power of persuasion automatically afforded by his position of authority. One experienced author has warned, "The counselor who habitually finds 'special cases' in which his 'superior' knowledge is used to influence his patients' decisions is not practicing as a counselor but rather as one who directs lives."[26]

It cannot be convincingly argued that persons at risk for HD have an *obligation* to forego the basic human right to reproduce. To sustain such an argument it would be necessary to prove an absolute certainty, or a very high probability, that an affected child would be born. Given our present state of knowledge, this is not possible with Huntington's disease. A person who is at risk may not have inherited the defective gene. Furthermore, HD is usually a late-onset disorder. Some people, even if they knew in advance that their child would be affected eventually, might still conclude that thirty-five or forty years of normal life is worth fifteen or twenty years with Huntington's disease. It is not a decision most of us would make, but none of us has a right to impose his view on others.

The Directive Argument

Counselors who espouse a more directive approach (that is, directive without being authoritarian) maintain that the non-directive argument is based on several questionable assumptions.

The first is that genuine "neutrality" actually exists. Feelings find expression not only through what we say and how we say it, but also through a complex repertoire of largely unconscious nonverbal communication. Directive counselors argue, therefore, that there is simply no way a counselor can avoid passing along his feelings to the counselee. Even if a counselor succeeds in hiding his convictions, his patient will probably try to guess at them. Rather than create such an unwholesome atmosphere, it is better to be open and honest. Admit at the outset that we are all fallible human beings, and remind the counselee that his decisions should not be made solely on the strength of the subjective opinions of the genetic counselor.[27] The goal is not to "direct" people toward a specific decision, but to help them understand *all* aspects of the problem. According to its advocates, this counseling is not so much *directive* as it is *guidance-oriented*.

A second questionable assumption in the nondirective argument is that all human beings are created equal and enjoy an equal right to determine their own destiny. The idea that all men are created equal sounds good in the Declaration of Independence, but it is obviously incorrect from a genetic point of view. A child born with Tay-Sachs disease is not "created equal" to a normal, healthy child. A person who inherits the gene for Huntington's disease is not born genetically equal to the vast majority of the population who will go through life never even knowing that the disease exists. Reproductive decisions rest ultimately with the parents, but those at risk for serious genetic disorders should not be led to believe that they are no different from anyone else.

In response to the argument that the unborn have a right to life, guidance-oriented counselors suggest that there should be a reasonable assurance of a healthy life. If we know before birth, or even before conception, that a child will either have a serious disease or be at very high risk for one, then we have an obligation to the unborn child and to society to prevent that individual from being subjected, through no choice of its own, to years of suffering. One authority has written, "In recent years, the feeling has grown among both physicians and the general public that we must be concerned not simply with ensuring the birth of a baby, but of one who will not be a liability to society, to its parents, and to itself. The 'right to be born' is becoming qualified by another right: to have a reasonable chance of a happy and useful life."[28]

Most parents would not hesitate to terminate a pregnancy if a disease like Tay-Sachs were diagnosed. What is the point of bringing into the world a baby who will suffer terribly and surely die within three or four years? (Of course, some people are resolutely opposed to terminating a pregnancy under any circumstances.)

The problem becomes infinitely more complex when we consider Huntington's disease. The Tay-Sachs example is clearly defined. We know before the pregnancy is well advanced that the fetus has Tay-Sachs, and we know the terrible consequences that will follow almost immediately if the baby is born. This is not true of Huntington's disease. We cannot say before or even after birth whether a baby carries the gene for the disorder, nor do we know how severe the symptoms will be if the gene has been inherited. We *do* know that symptoms probably will not begin to appear until the person has lived thirty-five or more years.

Many of us would agree that "society can legitimately expect protection from situations in which a person with HD . . . could place others at unusual risk."[29] In other words, most people (but not everyone) would agree that a person who *already has* HD should refrain from having children. When a woman who definitely has Huntington's disease becomes pregnant, we know with certainty that the baby will inherit a 50 percent risk for the disease if the pregnancy is brought to term. But what about someone who knows only that he or she is at risk for the disease? Should that person be given the same advice that would be offered to someone who actually has the disease? Some counselors would say definitely not. Others argue that guidance against procreation should be given because, even in these circumstances, the risk is too high.

Advocates of guidance-oriented counseling maintain that, at the very least, counselors have a responsibility to discuss all these issues, societal as well as personal, with the counselee. To do less is to deprive the individual of knowledge and understanding that are necessary to make a truly informed decision. Some counselors who believe themselves to be neutral are not even aware of some of the broader and more difficult issues. They make their job easier by "sticking to the simple facts," but they do nothing to help their patients appreciate the many subtle and subjective factors that are relevant in making vital decisions.

Resolving the Conflict

If nondirective counselors feel that they are ethically bound to remain strictly neutral, and advocates of a more guidance-oriented approach say that there is no neutrality, where does the conscientious counselor find a workable middle ground? F. Clarke Fraser points out that most counselors are neither strictly neutral nor categorically directive:

> Most counselors would refrain from directly telling the counselee what to do, but most would at least talk the matter over and point out the various factors that might be considered. Often the counselee will, after discussion, ask what the counselor would do if he were in the same situation. [A counselor might then] go so far as to say that although it is impossible to extrapolate himself entirely into the counselee's situation, since he is not the counselee, he thinks he would probably take a certain course of action.[30]

Some proponents of nondirective counseling would argue that this is going too far, but Fraser contends that the counselor is doing nothing more than surgeons do routinely when they recommend an elective operation. People come to counselors for advice and they are entitled to get it.[31] They can then make their own decision on how to use it.

No matter what that decision is, though, the counselor should try to remain supportive. Certainly a counselor should not show disappointment if he has offered advice which the counselee has rejected. This is particularly true when a decision to have a child is reached. The counselor may feel that a person who is at risk for HD should not have children. If a couple then decide otherwise, it is not the role of the counselor (or anyone else) to make them feel as if they have done something wrong. Under such circumstances, "genetic counseling" comes dangerously close to being a synonym for advice *not* to have children. Questions regarding human life are not to be reduced to comparative statistics or dollars and cents "burden" arguments. By what standard can anyone measure forty years without Huntington's disease and fifteen years with it against not being born at all? Marjorie Guthrie, who knew the sufferings of her folk singer husband better than anyone other than Woody himself, has asked if people would prefer that such a talented man had never existed.[32] Anyone who has ever loved a person at risk for Huntington's disease knows exactly what she means.

Another view has been persuasively put by John S. Pearson, a clinical psychologist in Wichita, Kansas. Dr. Pearson has concluded that "more people are happier longer when the decision against reproduction is made at the outset of the childbearing years." He found that, even among couples who lived beyond the usual age of onset without showing any symptoms of HD, "these individuals have remained happy with their adopted children or in their childless state, wasting no regrets over the fact that children they might have had would almost certainly be free of the hereditary taint." Among those at risk who went ahead and had children of their own, Pearson reported that in some cases

> the decision to have children was followed months or years later by the realization that symptoms of Huntington's disease were developing, that science had not found an answer, and that the children were subject to the 50% probability. In such instances a depressive reaction is commonly observed, not only in the affected individual but in his or her spouse, which is most pitiable and most difficult to treat. It is in experience of this kind that I base the flat assertion, persons at 50% risk of developing Huntington's disease should not have children.[33]

And so the debate continues. The genetic counselor may long for definitive answers and wish that the issues were not so complex and ambiguous. The way forward will become less difficult as scientific research improves our knowledge of the disease. Development of a reliable predictive test would be a major aid for genetic counseling, although the existence of such a test would also pose some complicated problems.[34] Until such a test, or more effective management tools, become available, the counselor's chief responsibility is to help people appreciate the complexity of the disease and facilitate their adjustment to it.

CONCLUSION

In 1977 the U.S. Commission for the Control of Huntington's Disease and Its Consequences summarized the objectives of genetic counseling for HD. Counselors should provide the counselee with accurate and detailed information with respect to: (1) basic genetic principles and the risks for HD, (2) the natural history of the disease, including early signs and progression, (3) the importance of autopsies when the diagnosis is uncertain, (4) treatment possibilities, (5) occupational and physical therapy services and limitations, (6) reproductive options, (7) varieties of care, either at home or in a hospital or nursing home, and the financial costs and insurance coverage each entails, (8) research potential: new leads, hopes, limitations, (9) legal and ethical problems of HD, (10) anticipation of possible social, sexual, career, financial, and other problems, and the provision of a referral network for future counseling and assistance.[35]

Counselors are acutely aware that their options for coping with incurable genetic disorders like Huntington's disease are severely limited. But the counselor faces an important responsibility precisely because the alternatives are so limited. The importance of exploiting fully the available options and support possibilities becomes obvious. Part of the counselor's job is to help the HD family discover where they can turn for tangible assistance.

One author has concluded that "in few areas of genetic counseling is the role of the counselor more psychotherapeutically oriented than in his work with patients from families with Huntington's chorea and similar progressive hereditary neurodegenerative disorders."[36] Psychotherapeutic counseling is a continuing process. Extensive and careful follow-up is as important as it is neglected in counseling HD families. Few people can make an optimal adjustment to something as serious as Huntington's disease after only one or two visits with a doctor or genetic counselor. General practitioners engaged in this type of counseling may find it difficult to chart a schedule of continuous contact with the HD family. But the importance of long-term counseling that is extended to all members of the family must not be overlooked. The physician-patient relationship is expanded to a physician-family relationship by the very nature of the disease.[37] Even after the family has made its initial adjustments to the disorder, follow-up interviews should be scheduled at least twice yearly. In this way the counselor can reinforce information already given, assess changes in attitude, and provide additional services where needed.[38]

A consensus will probably never be reached on what is the best approach to genetic counseling. But commonsense generalizations are a good beginning. Counselors should be patient, honest, and understanding. They should strive to communicate information about the disorder in a way that helps the counselee's adjustment process. They should encourage dialogue as a means of assessing the counselee's attitude and comprehension of vital information. They should be good listeners. They must be willing to devote the time and effort necessary to help each individual "work through" his or her particular relationship to the disorder. Counselors must respect confidentiality, but they should also take proper steps to inform people who may be unaware that they are at risk for a serious hereditary disorder.

Finally, the shoulders of the genetic counselor should be broad enough to carry the burden of unjustified accusation. When dealing with a condition like Huntington's disease, the counselor, be he family doctor or specialist, may sometimes act as a very useful lightning conductor to direct volatile emotions away from the family. When an individual or family is looking for a way to release anger or guilt, the counselor may be the most convenient target. As long as the counselor has done his or her best, this reaction can be absorbed with an appreciation of the acute human distress which prompts such behavior. The counselor's satisfaction must come from his knowledge that he has done his best to help the patient and the family.[39]

5

Management

I cared for my son at home as long as possible, then placed him in a rest home. He left his room one evening to get something to help him sleep. The nurses put him back in his room and locked it with a coat hanger from the outside. He fell to the floor and, after a time, managed to crawl to his bed and pull himself on it. One of the nurses told me that she and two of the other nurses watched him through an outside window. . . .

On November 5, 1975, Mrs. Suzan Smith died quietly in a nursing home in Atlanta, Georgia. She was fifty-eight years old. The cause of death was officially listed as Huntington's disease, but Suzan Smith actually suffocated when her emaciated body slipped between the mattress and a bedrail of the cot that had been the center of her world for more than two years. For most of that time, she suffered alone. Family and friends visited less and less frequently until she rarely received any visitors at all.

For forty years Suzan lived a normal, happy life. Then she began to feel continuously nervous and emotionally upset. She sought the advice of local doctors. Her symptoms grew worse, but none of the doctors could identify the source of her problem. Some of her friends said it was menopause. A neighbor who did not like her complained that Mrs. Smith was "just a bitchy old hypochondriac." Although they never said it openly, some of her doctors came to the same conclusion. They wished that she would quit pestering them. Several doctors prescribed placebos and sent her a bill they hoped would make her think twice before bothering them again.

Over a ten-year period, Suzan sought help from thirty-one different doctors. The combined service fees exceeded $36,000. Finally, she saw a heart specialist who knew enough about genetic disorders to suspect Huntington's disease. A careful search of Suzan's family history revealed that HD had existed in the family for several generations. It had been consistently misdiagnosed as schizophrenia. Huntington's disease had never been mentioned, and no one in the family knew anything about it. They were unaware that there was any connection between the sufferings of one generation and the next. Occasionally someone speculated that a "form of insanity" might run in the family, but that was all.[1]

The tragic story of Suzan Smith is not unique. In another case, a fifty-five-year-old woman in Colorado was declared mentally incompetent and committed to a state hospital, where she received repeated electric shock treatments. Her condition grew rapidly worse until her weight fell to only fifty-seven pounds. She was transferred to a private hospital, but remained completely helpless until she died a year later. Shortly before she died, the diagnostic error was discovered. She did not suffer from paranoid schizophrenia, as first thought, but from Huntington's disease.

Anyone familiar with the history of Huntington's disease knows that case studies like these could be listed almost indefinitely. The testimony taken in 1976–77 by the U.S. Commission for the Control of Huntington's Disease and Its Consequences provides ample documentation.[2] Many families touched by HD are desperate. They feel "almost totally deprived of support from any branch of society."[3] Their situation is poorly understood by doctors. Suggested treatment often does more harm than good. They can't get insurance. General hospitals won't take an HD patient. Nursing homes isolate them and "sometimes let them starve or choke." Relatives and former friends abandon them. There seems to be no place for the chronically ill. Reviewing the Commission's *Report*, one observer concluded: "In every piece of public testimony, the indictment of long-term care facilities for patients with Huntington's disease is clear. There are few even adequate facilities available . . . [and an] appalling lack of graded facilities for those with moderate disabilities."[4]

The failure to provide satisfactory institutional care for the chronically ill and neurologically handicapped is only part of the problem. The needs of these patients have been consistently overlooked in the provision of all health-related services. In countries without programs of comprehensive national health insurance, many needy families may be unable to afford the most basic care. The plea in the previous chapter for effective genetic counseling is pointless if low-income families are required to pay a substantial fee to the doctor or counselor.

The Commission's *Report* on Huntington's disease cited the need for "a program that permits flexibility in the range of services, facilities, and personnel to supply the physical and emotional needs of chronically ill patients over the long course of the disease. . . . The level of care should range from minimal once-a-week housecleaning services or a daily telephone call, to the fully protected environment and skilled care needed by a patient at the end stages of illness."[5]

Management of chronic degenerative disorders like Huntington's disease requires a continuum of services by a team of health care professionals. The objection is often raised that this is too expensive. But a team, properly utilized, can work in support of many doctors and several institutions, providing consultation and care for a large number of patients. The services of a trained geneticist, neurologist, social worker, psychiatrist, nurse, nutritionist, and physical, speech, or music therapist are not required all the time by every patient. The problem is that, under present circumstances, many patients do not benefit from the services of any of these people. Inadequate financial resources is the most common excuse for perpetuating an inferior care system, but the real reason is more commonly a lack of imagination, enterprise, and boldness on the part of administrators who should be exploring new ways to meet the pressing needs of chronically ill patients. The team approach to continuing care receives more detailed attention at the conclusion of this chapter.

DRUG THERAPY

When most people think about the management of any disease, they are likely to focus immediately on drugs. Treatment of complex, neurological disorders like Huntington's disease may evoke the image of a nurse making the rounds twice daily with a platter full of pills. Our society is preoccupied with drugs. We are encouraged to believe that all of our problems, from serious illness to lovesick loneliness, can be solved instantly by simply "popping a pill."

One of the most common questions asked about Huntington's disease is whether a miracle drug exists which can cure, check, or reverse the disorder. When people learn that there is no such drug, they then want to know how long it will be before one is developed. It is essential, therefore, to stress at the outset that there is no "miracle cure" for Huntington's disease. No available drug can reverse the process of brain cell deterioration.[6] There *are* drugs which can control some of the symptoms associated with Huntington's disease. The chorea (involuntary muscle movement) can be reduced in most patients. Drug therapy can also assist in the control of emotional disorders in some patients. But no drug can reverse the progressive intellectual deterioration, and all drugs must be administered with great care to avoid harmful side effects.

One of the reasons drug therapy is of limited use in Huntington's disease is that we still incompletely understand the root cause of the disorder. Since the exact mechanism that triggers the onset of the disease is not known, it is impossible to attack the problem at its point of origin. This is why doctors speak only in terms of "managing" the disease. Until researchers learn more about what actually causes HD, opening the possibility of curative treatment, doctors can only concentrate on alleviating symptoms and improving the care of individual patients. It is always possible, of course, that a highly effective drug could be discovered before the disease is fully understood. It is also possible that scientists may one day unravel the fundamental cause of HD and still face some years of work before they can cure the disease.

There is no single drug which doctors routinely use for patients with Huntington's disease. Certain classes of drugs have proven helpful, and these are discussed in a general way below. This discussion of drug therapy is *not* intended as a clinical guide. It is designed to give the general reader some idea of the types of drugs often used in the management of Huntington's disease, why they are used, and what they do. Readers who are personally concerned about a particular patient should seek the advice of a doctor, preferably a neurologist or other specialist with experience in the treatment of Huntington's disease. If a specialist is not known, referrals and assistance can be obtained from most major hospitals or from volunteer Huntington's disease organizations (see listings in appendix 2).

Drug therapy for genetic disorders is based on the basic physiological processes at work in these disorders. All genetic diseases stem from some alteration in the gene or DNA molecule, which may produce either an excess or deficiency of certain chemicals required to keep the body functioning properly. Drug intervention may be directed toward reducing an excess of unwanted substances; or the goal may be to increase the level of substances in inadequate supply; or it may be necessary to try to replace vital substances which, through some genetic malfunction, are missing entirely.

The ultimate answer, of course, would be to correct the underlying gene defect at the source of the problem.[7] The possibility of such "genetic engineering" is receiving considerable attention in research centers throughout the world. We are now at the brink of a revolution in the science of genetics, a period of discovery fraught with great promise and great peril. Gerald Edelman, molecular biologist at New York's Rockefeller University, has noted that humanity is approaching an understanding of the innermost secrets of the human cell. In 1979 he said, "After years of slogging through the mud, we will soon be flying in the air. . . . We are in a predicament about certain diseases, but once we thoroughly understand the human cell, it will be like walking through fields of clover to treat them."[8]

Unfortunately, the fields of clover are not an immediate prospect for those who must live daily with the reality of Huntington's disease. Dominantly inherited conditions may yield one day to genetic manipulation but, until then, they remain among the most difficult to treat comprehensively and effectively. This is especially true of chronic, degenerative disorders like Huntington's disease, because they involve a broad and variable range of physical, emotional, and intellectual symptoms.

In a sense, all drug treatment for Huntington's disease is

experimental, because we do not know enough about the basic biochemical mechanisms at work in the disease to know exactly what a drug is doing for, or to, a patient. Treatment of this type is said to be "empirical" because it relies on experience and observation for validation of its effectiveness. Partly for this reason, a wide variety of drugs have been, and continue to be, used in the treatment of Huntington's disease. Sometimes ignorance, excessive zeal to try a new drug, or the eager wish to relieve the suffering of a patient has led to the prescription and continued use of drugs which were inappropriate and did more harm than good.

For many years, sedatives, particularly barbiturates like phenobarbital, were most commonly used in the treatment of Huntington's disease.[9] During the 1950s a new class of drugs known as neuroleptics came into common use. A *neuroleptic* is a drug which "by its characteristic actions and effects is useful in the treatment of mental disorders."[10] Neuroleptics commonly used in the management of HD include chlorpromazine, haloperidol, perphenazine, and tetrabenazine. The most widely used drugs for the treatment of HD are the phenothiazines and butyrophenones. These are neuroleptics which are believed to act by blocking dopamine receptors in the brain.[11]

For reasons not fully understood, some drugs work for some HD patients and not for others. Sometimes the physician will experiment carefully with several alternative drugs until he finds those which are most helpful to a particular patient.

Care should be taken not to begin drug therapy too early or rely on it too much. The severe symptoms and progressive nature of the disease may invite overzealous treatment. Dr. Ira Shoulson of Rochester University in New York has warned that "a polypharmacy approach should be avoided."[12] The patient's response to the introduction of any drug must be closely monitored for side effects. There are many possible disadvantages in the routine use of neuroleptic drugs for patients with Huntington's disease. One common problem associated with the frequent use of these drugs is a marked increase in depression. It is unwise to prescribe for HD patients, who are already likely to suffer from depression, drugs that may make them more depressed. Some experts believe that careless use of these drugs has sometimes been sufficient to tip the balance and cause patients to commit suicide.[13]

PSYCHIATRIC CARE

The appearance of psychiatric symptoms may predate the diagnosis of Huntington's disease by a considerable span of years. One study of the sociopsychiatric characteristics of 102 Huntington's disease patients yielded some disturbing findings. Self-aggression was common. One patient committed suicide, ten others made suicidal attempts, thirteen patients mutilated themselves, and there were nineteen cases of alcoholism. In twenty-three (38 percent) of the married patients, the marriages broke up and divorce or separation occurred. Criminality occurred in eighteen patients; the offenses included assault, offenses against property, and cruelty to children.[14]

Even when psychiatric symptoms do not involve psychotic or criminal behavior, adequate management can be difficult to achieve. Dr. Shoulson has written, "The psychiatric management of HD patients is difficult and often unrewarding despite its critical importance to both patient and his family."[15] Some of the personal and family problems are illustrated in the following serious, but not atypical, case reported from the Creedmoor Institute in New York:

A 41-year-old white housewife was referred for study to Creedmoor Institute in August, 1959, by a local psychiatrist. Her mother had died at 71, having had Huntington's disease for 29 years. [In 1953] there had been onset of diminution in interest, slowing of activity, and fatigue. She was at that time found to be mildly hypertensive. Hyperkinesia appeared four years later, manifested by mild choreoid activity of feet or legs, extension-flexion movement of the trunk and inability to sit still, the latter especially noticeable during attendance at church. Gradually, depression appeared. Activities became effortful. She was bored with work, could not force herself to do housework or former hobbies, and began to lie down several hours each afternoon. With progression of the illness, she said that she wished she were dead, hated to return to the house after trips, stopped laughing altogether and smiled only rarely. It was soon necessary for her husband to bathe her, to help her dress, and to comb her hair. She began to remain bedfast most of the day due to weakness, became occasionally incontinent of urine and feces, retained food and saliva in her mouth for long periods, and had to be reminded to keep herself clean. . . .[16]

This case clearly illustrates the variety of symptoms that signal the onset of Huntington's disease. Slowing of interest and activity, involuntary muscle movement, loss of attention to personal appearance, and a change of personality all may indicate the presence of the disorder. Other signs might include irritability, intolerance, lapses of memory, emotional outbursts, and depression.

For the housewife in this case, depression became a serious problem, presumably even before she was diagnosed as having Huntington's disease. For obvious reasons, depression is one of the most common symptoms among HD patients. It is difficult to face a bleak future without becoming depressed. This is one of the reasons why HD patients need to be reassured that, with effort, their productive life may be extended for many years. Psychiatric care obviously goes beyond the prescription of drugs.

Doctors are not certain to what extent the depression associated with Huntington's disease is *reactive* and to what extent it is *endogenous*. Depression may occur merely as a reaction to the presence or threat of HD, or it may be a product of actual biochemical changes in the brain. In most cases, it is probably some combination of both. Reactive depression should be more amenable to treatment than a depressed state which results from biochemical changes. It may be that much more of the depression associated with Huntington's disease is reactive than experts have believed.[17] Traditionally, HD patients contemplating both their future and their present state of care have had ample reason to get depressed. After all, plenty of perfectly healthy people with no risk for hereditary disease and no particular reason to feel bad manage to get depressed.

Reactive depression in Huntington's disease can often be alleviated, to some extent at least, by careful counseling and supportive therapy. The presence of severe depression or psychotic behavior in some HD patients may require more intensive therapy, however. Dr. Shoulson has written, "Some patients have responded to anti-depressant agents; in this regard, the tricyclic antidepressants are preferable."[18] In some instances, significant improvement may come from this form of therapy. After a month, the specialists reported marked progress in the forty-one-year-old housewife discussed above:

> ... her mood had improved markedly, her appetite had increased, and she had begun to take interest in former activities. ... Mood and behavioral improvements continued through the fall with family and friends recognizing 'amazing change' from the previous summer. She returned to baking cakes and pies, no longer required assistance in bathing, dressing, or toilet care and took only occasional naps. Weight gradually increased.[19]

In this particular case, drug therapy produced a favorable result, although there were some side effects (an increase in blood pressure and a worsening of chorea). The woman's relationship to other members of the family was much improved, along with her ability to look after herself. The doctors treating her realized that any case of Huntington's disease involves the whole family. The person who actually has the disease may not be the only one who is in need of counseling or psychiatric assistance. It is good for other members of the family to be aware of this and seek help when they feel the pressures accumulating. Ignoring one's own needs may lead to exhaustion or emotional breakdown, and so deprive the HD patient of his or her primary care provider.[20]

A CREATIVE ATTACK THROUGH OCCUPATIONAL, PHYSICAL, RECREATIONAL, AND MUSICAL THERAPY

Self-esteem is critical to the mental health and well-being of each of us. If we are "down on" ourselves, convinced that we are inferior or a burden to society, we will inevitably suffer from all sorts of mental and physical problems. Not surprisingly, HD patients are especially likely to have bad feelings about themselves. When the patient's capabilities are restricted due to illness and he is given no opportunity to express himself, his sense of personal value may decline so much that he eventually loses the will to live.

There is ample clinical evidence to suggest that at least part of the deterioration in Huntington's disease is linked to the environmental deprivation associated with the patient's restricted existence.[21] The primary goal of various forms of nondrug therapy is to break down the environmental barriers and expand the patient's opportunities for self-realization and fulfillment. Occupational, physical, recreational, and musical therapy are among the tools used to achieve these ends. Time, effort, and plenty of patience are needed, but the results can be extraordinarily rewarding.

These forms of therapy do not require specialized training in all cases. For example, regular exercise—one of the most useful therapeutic tools in existence—is especially effective for people whose bodies are forced to cope with a degenerative illness.[22] Patients with Huntington's disease and related disorders are often stereotyped as "helpless incurables," and then confined in ways which prevent them from demonstrating that they are far from helpless. When given the opportunity, they may prove perfectly capable of doing exercises and accomplishing certain tasks which were believed beyond their reach. This improves their self-image, makes them more active, fosters new goals in life, and expands the opportunity for contacts with other people. Similarly, the pursuit of hobbies—arts, crafts, sports, games, etc.—can offer a patient new interests and challenges, as well as the promise of social interaction and a chance to achieve and create.[23]

Music therapy is one area of Huntington's disease care which is seriously neglected. Listening to good music has a soothing effect, and music therapists report that HD patients are capable of active musical expression. This may include singing or, in less serious cases, dancing or the playing of a simple musical instrument.[24]

The potential for improvement among HD patients who are given new opportunities is well illustrated by one program carried out by a doctor and an occupational therapist working jointly. Phyllis Borgelt and Dr. Thomas Linde worked with a number of patients in the advanced stages of Huntington's disease. None of these patients could walk. They could not convey themselves to bed or toilet. Some could no longer feed themselves. They were thought to be incapable of creative activities.

Borgelt and Linde decided to try to make amateur weavers of the whole group. Small, ordinary wooden looms were used. They were strung with heavy nylon material to prevent breakage. Patients who were apprehensive or reluctant to weave were simply encouraged to do what they could. Rather than make demands, the therapists praised the slightest progress, stressing possibilities and potential. Sometimes a therapist intervened to help a patient over a particularly difficult patch or to complete the final tying of the rug. Completed rugs were displayed in the hospital, and patients were reminded that many people would see and appreciate their handiwork. Some patients also learned how to fashion ashtrays and trivets using ceramic tiles and other materials. Finished items were sometimes given, with obvious and justifiable pride, as gifts to relatives or friends. As patients proved their abilities to themselves and to their families, consulting psychologists noted that the specter of the disease became less threatening and the bond among family members stronger.[25]

Occupational therapy can mean many things. It is not simply weaving rugs and it does not come into play only when the patient is seriously disabled. It is wise to begin thinking about alternative occupational and physical activities long before the disease reaches its final stages. Sometimes alternative interests are most required when the disorder is in its early or middle stages. This is particularly true when the customary breadwinner is forced to alter or abandon his career. The breadwinner may be either the husband or the wife. In either case, the loss of that role may prompt a difficult period of adjustment. Loss of a job or professional status can be a serious blow to the self-esteem of anyone. It may be especially hard for men, whose role as the primary providers of income is still traditional in most families. Men who have been conditioned all their lives by sex role stereotypes may limit their own usefulness by refusing to exchange roles with their wives. Some people, both men and women, are so involved with their work that they never develop alternative interests and hobbies which can help fill the void created by loss of that work.

The experience of one family in Sydney, Australia, provides an instructive example of smooth adjustment when Huntington's disease began to appear. The father in this family had a thriving career when the first symptoms of the disorder became apparent. After a few years he could no longer maintain his position, despite his employer's willingness to reduce the demands of the job. When this happened, his wife took a full-time job, and he assumed primary responsibility for the household duties. He vacuumed and scrubbed the floors, dusted, did the shopping, washed the clothes, and did most of the cooking. This role reversal was not without its difficulties because, like most men, he had been conditioned by the sexist labeling of household activities as "women's work." He was also subjected to curious and disapproving stares from the public when he ambled, somewhat unsteadily, to the local shops. He was humiliated once when a store manager mistook him for drunk and telephoned the police. Uniformed officers escorted him from the store and drove him home where one of his children managed to explain the situation to their satisfaction.

Despite occasional setbacks, the man in this family adjusted rapidly to his new role in life. Household duties were physically demanding but within his capabilities. His contribution to family welfare proved vital to his self-esteem, and he received assistance and frequent expressions of appreciation from his wife and children. His willingness to take over many of her former duties helped his wife to cope with the enormous demands placed on her when she entered the workforce. She realized that she was more fortunate than some women in a similar situation, who are required to assume simultaneous roles as breadwinner, primary care provider, household administrator, and mother.

Although few, if any, studies have been done on the subject, it appears that women usually manage better than men to assume added responsibility when a mate is chronically ill.[26] Most men whose wives have Huntington's disease do not face a transition but a continuation as breadwinner; they may employ professional household and nursing assistance. Yet men often seem to feel excessively burdened by the new demands. Perhaps women have both the experience and the strength to deal more effectively than men with prolonged crisis situations.[27] It may also be true that many men are so protected by loving mothers and wives that they become disoriented when called upon to manage for themselves while caring for someone else.

NURSING CARE

Nurses are the front-line troops in the battle to manage

Huntington's disease. The medical specialist may formulate the drug regimen and guide treatment, but it is the nurse who deals with the patient hour after hour and day after day. In some cases this can be a frustrating, even dangerous, experience.

Few nurses have been adequately trained to deal with the unique care problems posed by a disorder as complex and difficult as Huntington's disease. Sometimes overworked nurses are so intimidated by the disease that they grow angry and vindictive toward the patient. They come to see their job as little more than keeping the patient alive and quiet. Watching through an outside window while a disabled patient crawls to his bed is inexcusable, but it may be as much the product of fear and a sense of futility as it is negligence.

A nurse's negative attitude only adds to the serious problems already faced by the person who has the disease. Nurses should bear in mind that most HD patients are "frightened, frustrated individuals who need support, encouragement and respect as much as they need physical care."[28] By gearing the daily program toward maintaining as much of the patient's independence as possible for as long as possible, nurses can very effectively improve the patient's morale. This is an extraordinarily important contribution. The following suggestions are guided by the principle of preserving the HD patient's independence.

First, the patient's total environment should be planned and structured to minimize the threat of injury. Self-injury is a major problem for any patient with severe involuntary muscle movements (nurses must also exercise care that they are not themselves harmed by the patient's uncontrolled flailing movements). Beds, chairs, and floors may require padding. Foam rubber with removable, washable covers is useful for beds, chairs, and re-straining devices. If a patient with extreme movements is in danger of overturning a special chair, such as a geriatric chair, secure the device temporarily to a solid piece of furniture. Restraints should only be used when absolutely necessary to protect the patient's safety. They should be adjusted and changed regularly. Some patients with advanced symptoms may require minimal restraint to keep them from toppling out of a chair, but a patient should *never* be restrained for long periods. Rather than restrain the patient, the nurse should try to adjust the environment. Research is currently under way in Australia to design an adjustable chair that will make the use of restraint unnecessary.

Make the environment cheerful as well as safe. Pictures and flowers always brighten a room. If there is no money available for these things, contact the nearest Huntington's disease organization for advice and help.

Special care must be exercised at meals. Persons with advanced HD symptoms are often in danger of choking, so it is a good idea to include a sucking machine as part of ward equipment. Nurses should be well trained in the proper medical procedures in the event of choking or aspiration problems. Weight loss is also a chronic problem; double portions of a soft diet plus between-meal high-protein supplements and frequent snacks may be necessary. Tea, coffee, and hot food should be cooled to prevent burns from spills.

Every daily activity can be accompanied by some form of verbal communication. Patients with advanced symptoms may not be able to speak clearly. But the inability to form words does not imply an inability to comprehend them. Many people with Huntington's disease are deeply frustrated because, while they fully comprehend events around them, they are unable to make known their needs and opinions. To alleviate this situation, one group of nurses made a large chart with pictures illustrating various recognizable needs—food, drink, wash, toilet—that made it easy for the patient to indicate what she wanted. Recognizing that their patient's inability to speak clearly did not mean she was unable to *understand* speech, these nurses also went out of their way to communicate with her: "Whenever we had free time we would talk and read to her as she lacked the concentration to read or entertain herself, and it also meant that we kept some form of communication open, even if it was mainly one way."[29] Such a spirit, one that is enlightened by both empathy and practicality, is the best that the nursing profession can be expected to offer.

Detailed suggestions for the care of HD patients at home, prepared by the Department of Health, State of New York, in conjunction with the Committee to Combat Huntington's Disease, are contained in appendix 1.

THE TEAM APPROACH TO HD MANAGEMENT

Huntington's disease is best managed by a team of experienced professionals. This chapter has focused on the role of the neurologist, psychiatrist, therapist, and nurse. There should be other members of the team as well. The social worker, nutritionist, speech therapist, and minister, priest, or rabbi also have an important contribution to make.

The team approach to continuous care is receiving attention in many countries—Canada, England, nations of continental Europe, and elsewhere. In Australia, for example, the Huntington's Disease Care Centre at Mary's Mount in Balwyn, Victoria, is the first facility of its type in the world. When it began receiving its first patients in 1980, it teamed the services of neurologists, geneticists, social workers, nurses, researchers, volunteer drivers, etc. In Australia, more than most other modern countries, such desperately needed work suffers from the failure of the government to allocate sufficient funds. Most of the financial support for Mary's Mount has come from the Wesley Central Mission. The bus that transports day patients to and from the center was donated by a private benefactor. But despite financial constraints, Mary's Mount promises to set an example of what the collective approach can accomplish in HD care.

In the United States, the Commission for the Control of Huntington's Disease has outlined a team approach to the management of HD and related disorders. The Commission foresees "Centers Without Walls"—clinical and research facilities which serve, among other things, as the administrative base for outreach teams designed to provide information, training, treatment, and care for patients and their families. The agency to administer these centers would be the National Institute of Neurological and Communicative Disorders and Stroke (NINCDS).[30]

As founder and president emeritus of the Committee to Combat Huntington's Disease, Marjorie Guthrie has put together a plan for a Diagnostic and Referral Center to serve as a model for a Center Without Walls. The plan outlines the essential personnel and services required to sustain a program of continuous care for patients with chronic, degenerative disorders. (See figure 5.1.)

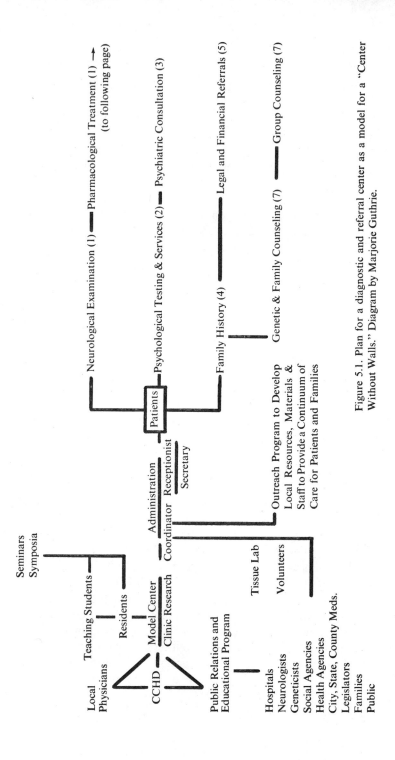

Figure 5.1. Plan for a diagnostic and referral center as a model for a "Center Without Walls." Diagram by Marjorie Guthrie.

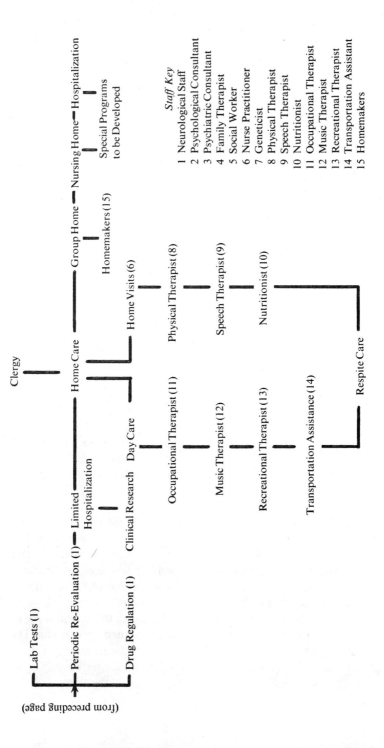

6

Predictive Testing and Early Detection

Perhaps the most frustrating aspect of the disease is the "not knowing who will be afflicted and when." Having lived on an "at risk" basis for 40 years is such a mental strain that even if one "escapes" the direct effects, he suffers indirectly for the major part of his lifespan.

One of the primary goals of Huntington's disease research is the development of a simple, safe, and reliable test to detect the presence of the defective gene long before the appearance of overt symptoms of the disorder.[1] At present, *no such test exists.* There is no proven method of predicting who carries the gene for Huntington's disease and who does not before symptoms are unmistakably present.

Development of an accurate predictive test might seem, at first thought, to be a way of conquering the disease. If such a test existed, those who returned a negative result (showing that they were free of the defective gene) could put their minds at ease and live normal lives. Those who returned a positive result (showing that they were carriers of the gene) would know well in advance of the onset of actual symptoms that they would eventually have to cope with Huntington's disease. Even though this would come as tragic news, it would at least give them time to prepare. The awful "not knowing" would be over. Vital decisions, such as whether or not to have children, would no longer be part of an agonizing guessing game.

Further reflection shows that the matter is not so simple, however. Problems raised by the prediction of a dominant genetic disorder of late onset are extraordinarily complex and riddled with ethical ambiguities.[2] This is particularly true if a predictive test is perfected in advance of a cure for the disease, as seems likely with Huntington's disease. Many types of predictive test are now under investigation, and they all present problems, even those which might be conducted *in utero* (prenatally) by some routine procedure such as amniocentesis.

Of course, if a reliable predictive test did exist, some people at risk for Huntington's disease might choose to forego it as long as the disease remained incurable. They might prefer to continue to live with a fifty-fifty risk rather than to chance learning that they definitely had the disease.

For those who took the test, if it were not proven to be absolutely accurate in every case, what would be done about false positive or false negative results? A false positive finding could have grievous consequences. What if a subject of such a test, informed of a positive result, on the strength of that finding decided not to marry, not to have children, not to pursue a professional career—only to be told years later, when he was very old and very healthy, that the test result had been in error? A false negative test could be even more tragic. A person who received false negative test results would live for years with the assurance that he was free of the defective gene, only to learn later—after having had many children, perhaps, or in the middle of a demanding career—that the test result had been incorrect. Even if a reliable test did emerge, it might have only short-term validity. A person who received a negative test result might have to be told, "It's negative for now, but come back in five years and check again."[3]

To make things even more complicated, predictive testing may not be simply a matter of positive or negative test results. Some predictive testing research has to do with probabilities. It is conceivable that a test could be developed which, while not giving an absolute answer, would modify the fifty-fifty risk. For example, a genetic linkage procedure might theoretically be developed which would indicate that one person is 95 percent likely to carry the gene for Huntington's disease while another person is only

10 percent likely to be a carrier. Genetic linkage will receive closer examination later in this chapter.

If we assume for a moment that a completely reliable predictive test did exist, the advantages for those found to be free of the defective gene are obvious. But what about the immediate and long-range consequences for those who were discovered to carry the gene? How would *you* react to being told that at some future time in your life it was absolutely certain you would develop a neurological disorder as serious as Huntington's disease? While some people might be able to adjust to this news reasonably well, others would react unpredictably, perhaps self-destructively.

Partly for this reason, some people might decide to take a predictive test only at a time when they were seriously contemplating having children. Their concern would be not so much for their own future as for the future of their children. But, even here, the problems do not end. Let us suppose, for example, that a predictive test indicated that a young married person did carry the gene for Huntington's disease, and that this person was emotionally strong enough to come to terms with the inevitability of his or her own fate. What about the question of having children? That the young person is a known carrier merely means that any offspring will inherit a fifty-fifty risk. It does not mean that each child will surely get the disease. Young people in this position would be better informed than their counterparts at present can be, but the fate of an unborn child would not be certain unless the fetus itself could be tested for the genetic defect.

PRENATAL PREDICTIVE TESTING

Many different genetic disorders can now be detected prenatally. Unfortunately, Huntington's disease is not yet one of them. But even if a prenatal test for HD existed, it would not solve all problems. If prospective parents discovered by means of such a test that their unborn child carried the gene for HD, what then? Should they opt for a therapeutic abortion? What about parents who are opposed to abortion? Even if the HD gene is present, the offspring may live thirty-five or forty years, perhaps longer, before any symptoms begin to appear. How are parents to weigh this prospect?

To these questions and others, there will never be easy answers. Still, if an accurate predictive test for Huntington's disease is developed, most experts would agree that the earlier in life it can be used, the better. Prenatal predictive tests have the advantage of offering an alternative—therapeutic abortion—which is obviously not available if the detection test can only be used after a person has been born. While promising work is being done toward developing a prenatal predictive test for HD, it cannot be assumed that a breakthrough is imminent. Significant advances have been made in recent years in detecting and treating recessive disorders, but the dominant diseases have proven far more difficult to crack. Part of the reason for this is that the recessive disorders tend toward a specific metabolic action in a localized part of the body, while the dominant diseases often involve a variety of biochemical changes at a number of different sites.[4]

The ability to detect the presence of a disease early in the fetal stage of development represents a major advance in medical genetics.[5] In the most common procedure, known as amniocentesis, a long, thin needle is inserted through the wall of the mother's abdomen and into the uterus. A local anaesthetic is used to desensitize the area where the needle is inserted. A sample of the amniotic fluid surrounding the fetus is withdrawn. The prospective mother is then ready to return home. The whole procedure is safe, simple, relatively painless, and highly reliable.

Over a period of several weeks, cells contained in the amniotic fluid sample taken from the mother are tested for chromosomal or other biochemical defects. If none appear, the fetus is presumed to be healthy. In most cases where amniocentesis is used, this is the happy result.[6] This would not be true, of course, if amniocentesis or some similar procedure could be used to detect Huntington's disease. Because the risk for the disease is so high, the number of positive tests would also be high. If either one of the parents were known to carry the defective gene, about one in every two pregnancies tested would yield a positive result.[7] This is one reason why many scientists believe it is urgent that a predictive test for HD be developed.

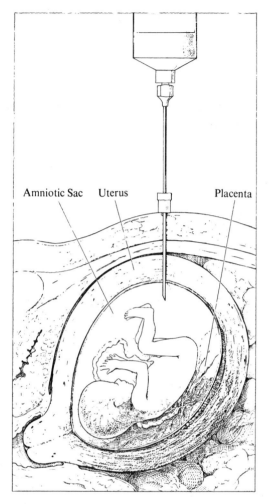

Amniotic Sac   Uterus   Placenta

Figure 6.1. Amniocentesis. A needle is inserted through a pregnant woman's abdominal wall to obtain fluid from the sac in which the fetus is suspended. Samples of this fluid, and of the cells floating in it, are used for the prenatal diagnosis of genetic disease. The illustration shows the fetus in the fifteenth week of pregnancy. This is the time at which amniocentesis is best performed, in part because the fluid has sufficient volume for the sample to be taken and in part because the completion of the tests of the fluid and its cells, two to four weeks after the fluid is sampled, leaves open to the prospective parents the choice of having the pregnancy ended if a severe disease is diagnosed. Many of the fetal abnormalities that can be detected by amniocentesis lead to crippling, life-shortening disorders. Huntington's disease, unfortunately, cannot yet be diagnosed by this procedure. From "Genetic Amniocentesis" by Fritz Fuchs. Copyright © 1980 by Scientific American, Inc. All rights reserved.

When amniocentesis yields a positive test result, several options are available. One is to terminate the pregnancy. Most people who undertake a monitored pregnancy plan to have a therapeutic abortion if tests indicate that the child will be born with a serious disease or disability. (Those who are resolutely opposed to abortion have no reason to monitor a pregnancy, in most cases.) But, quite aside from ethical questions surrounding abortion, legal barriers sometimes severely limit the individual's freedom of choice in the matter. Some Catholic countries outlaw abortion and disavow amniocentesis and prenatal diagnosis.

Among couples who will at least consider the option of abortion, the late onset characteristic of Huntington's disease raises additional problems. Many people would argue that it is one thing to terminate a pregnancy when a disease like Tay-Sachs is detected, but quite another where HD is concerned. Tay-Sachs, which can be detected by amniocentesis, is a condition in which the baby degenerates quickly, and never reaches maturity. This is not true of Huntington's disease. Most people who inherit the gene for HD will have three or four decades of healthy life before symptoms of the disease begin to appear. Even then, some HD patients will cope reasonably well for many years after the disorder has been diagnosed. Is abortion advisable under these circumstances? What is to be done when there is no way of knowing when the disease will appear or how serious it will be? Is it fair to gamble with the fate of the unborn child? By what standard is a judgment to be made in situations like this?

Even when amniocentesis is possible, there are problems involving time. Amniocentesis cannot be satisfactorily performed until at least twelve weeks of the pregnancy have elapsed, and fourteen weeks are preferable. Cells cultured from the amniotic fluid then require anywhere from two to four weeks for development and analysis, by which time the pregnancy may be into its eighteenth week. For both legal and medical reasons, a therapeutic abortion should be performed before the twentieth week of pregnancy. The twentieth week is well beyond the time when an abortion can safely be done by a dilatation and curettage. There are other means available, but they are more difficult and more subject to challenge on legal and ethical grounds.[8]

Weighing the rights of the prospective mother, the unborn child, and society-at-large can involve quite complicated ethical and legal questions. In December, 1978, for example, the New York Court of Appeals ruled that in certain circumstances physicians in that state could be held liable for the lifetime care of children born with some disorders which could have been detected prenatally. One case concerned a thirty-seven-year-old woman who was not advised by her doctor that the risk of bearing a child with Down's syndrome (mongolism) increases markedly when the mother passes the age of thirty-five. Her pregnancy was not monitored, and she gave birth to a girl affected by the disease. She sued, and the Court of Appeals found in her favor.[9]

Those who supported the New York court's decision concluded that it was based on careful medical reasoning which would help avoid tragic births. But some critics pointed out that doctors might be intimidated by the decision and be tempted to practice a form of "defensive medicine" by advising abortion rather than risking having to pay for the lifetime care of a handicapped child. The result could be the abortion of a baby that would have been healthy, as the only alternative to the threat of financial liability. At the very least, opponents argued, the decision would increase the number of tests administered during pregnancy and escalate malpractice insurance premiums. These new expenses would be passed on to the consumer in the form of further inflation of already high medical costs.[10]

If prenatal diagnosis reveals the presence of a disease or serious defect, there are other options besides abortion. These include: (1) prenatal treatment in the rare instances where this is technically possible; (2) bringing the pregnancy to term and assisting parents and child by means of whatever treatment is available for the condition; (3) bringing the pregnancy to term and leaving the family to cope with the condition as best they can; and (4) bringing the pregnancy to term and arranging for the adoption, foster care, or institutionalization of the child.

After studying the alternatives, one team of experts concluded, "Ethical considerations make it imperative to separate the fact of a positive diagnosis from the choice about the subsequent action. What parents and physicians should decide to do is not automatically dictated by the diagnosis, but ought to be shaped by their ethical and social views. . . . the lack of a moral consensus on abortion also makes it inappropriate to suggest that women have a moral (or 'medically indicated') obligation to undergo prenatal diagnosis."[11]

Of course, some people at risk for Huntington's disease would not want to have children even if a prenatal predictive test did exist and could assure them that only a healthy fetus would be carried to term. The knowledge that their children might have to face the difficulties of living with a chronically ill parent would be seen as reason enough, by some couples, for going childless.

This discussion of prenatal diagnosis is relevant for anyone concerned about what the future may hold in the area of predictive testing for Huntington's disease. The prenatal predictive procedures now used to detect disorders like Down's syndrome, Tay-Sachs, Cystinosis, Pompe syndrome, Gaucher's disease, Niemann-Pick disease, Hunter syndrome, Hurler syndrome, and many other (mostly recessive) disorders are *not* now possible for dominant conditions like Huntington's disease, but it is important to examine the special considerations raised by predictive testing in advance of its perfection. Some of the anticipated problems make it clear that development of a reliable predictive test, while very helpful, will not be a magic solution to the disease.

PRESYMPTOMATIC DETECTION*

If prenatal detection proves impossible, development of a predictive test which could be used before the reproductive years would at least enable persons at risk for Huntington's disease to determine their own situation before they decide whether or not to have children. Unfortunately, the quest to develop such a test is hampered by a variety of obstacles. For one thing, experimental tests require years of careful work and numerous repetitions to validate. Let us suppose, for example, that a research team did hit upon the perfect predictive test. How would they know it? Among persons known to be at risk for the disease, about half

* Strictly speaking, *presymptomatic* detection means identification of carriers of a disorder at any stage, including prenatal diagnosis, before the time symptoms begin to appear. As used here, however, the term applies to predictive testing which is done only after the subject is born.

would show a positive test result. This would not prove the validity of the test, however. Some of the results could turn out to be false. In order for a test to be proven accurate, the results must be verified repeatedly.

Because it takes so long to verify results, the medical journals are heavy with articles on promising preliminary research for predictive tests, but light on follow-up material which validates that research. One example in which follow-up data *were* recorded illustrates some of the problems inherent in research of this type.

Twenty-six persons at risk for Huntington's disease in Michigan took part in an electro-encephalographic (EEG) predictive test experiment in 1948. Nineteen of these people (73.1 percent) showed definite EEG abnormalities. The researchers concluded that twelve subjects with the greatest EEG abnormalities were likely to have inherited the gene for Huntington's disease. Eighteen years later, twenty-three of the twenty-six persons originally tested were contacted for a follow-up study. Of the twenty-three, eleven were still healthy and twelve showed symptoms of HD. But only five of these twelve were originally classified as likely to have the defective gene. Three had been classified as possibly having it and four as probably not having it. The follow-up study led to the conclusion that the original test was valueless for revealing the presence of HD presymptomatically.[12]

In this example, the follow-up study took place many years after the original test. In research of this nature, what is to be done during that long wait with the subjects who have been tested? The test is only experimental and may prove useless. But it is understandable that some people at risk for HD may not be able to maintain a scientific detachment about the whole thing. Can people who have a negative test result be blamed if they go away with a conviction that they are free of the disease? And what about those who return a positive result? Many of them are bound to conclude that they carry the gene. No amount of reassurance will convince everyone that the test is "for research purposes only."

The alternative to revealing the test result is to withhold that information. This is the usual practice. Subjects who volunteer for such tests are told at the outset that the project is experimental and the results will not be revealed. Most people go along with this. However, a number of researchers have had unhappy experiences with volunteers who have agreed to abide by these rules but later changed their minds and went to great lengths to obtain their test results. With so much at stake, this reaction is understandable. Nevertheless, it seriously complicates the already difficult problems associated with research projects designed to discover a reliable predictive test for Huntington's disease.

Most of these projects are based on the assumption that subtle changes occur in the person carrying the gene for the disease long before overt symptoms appear. If these changes do occur and a test is devised to detect them with precision, the means will be at hand to reliably predict the presence of the disease before it becomes manifest. A wide variety of experiments have been undertaken with this goal in mind. For some years now, researchers have worked with such things as psychological and language tests; fingerprint patterns; muscle response tests; spatial orientation tests; attention-span tests; the recording of subtle movements of the eyes, fingers, and tongue; and genetic linkage studies. Although such research has produced some promising clues, it has not yet resulted in a reliable predictive test.[13]

If the reader will bear with a brief, technical statement, studies have focused more recently on "skin fibroblast culture, electronic spin resonance on red cell membranes, tests of endocrine and hypothalamic function, computed axial tomography of the cerebral ventricles, *in vitro* responses to central nervous system antigens, and measurements of gamma-aminobutyric acid in the cerebrospinal fluid."[14] Here again, some of the initial findings have been encouraging, but much more needs to be done before any of these tests can be considered definitive. It would not be practical or useful to comment in detail on all these approaches, but several are worth closer examination because they illustrate some of the special problems involved in research for a predictive test.

One experimental approach grew from the observation that Huntington's disease exhibits biochemical changes which are opposite from those known to exist in Parkinson's disease. Drugs which work to control the symptoms of Parkinsonism often worsen the symptoms of Huntington's disease. Chief among these drugs is L-DOPA, and some researchers have tried to use it to detect the presence of HD presymptomatically.

In the early 1970s, scientists experimented with a predictive test predicated on the theory that persons at risk for HD who actually carry the defective gene will react to L-DOPA in ways fundamentally different from those who are at risk but do not carry the gene. Known as the "L-DOPA load test," the experiment assumed that administration of L-DOPA, by stimulating hypersensitive receptors in the cells of individuals who carried the gene, would temporarily elicit choreic movements long before those movements would otherwise become apparent.

In a 1972 test, thirty offspring of diagnosed HD patients were selected for trial, along with twenty-five control subjects who were not at risk for the disease. Everyone was given L-DOPA. Ten of the thirty persons at risk developed clear-cut facial and limb movements of the type usually seen in Huntington's disease. None of the twenty-five normal control subjects showed any movements. Once administration of L-DOPA was discontinued, the choreic movements disappeared from the ten people who were affected during the test. Follow-up data reported in 1980, eight years after the original test, revealed that "of the 10 subjects in whom transient chorea developed after exposure to levodopa [L-DOPA], five have since been found to have Huntington's disease, on the basis of subsequent development of chorea with or without behavioral changes. Of 20 patients at risk who had no chorea while receiving levodopa, one has since been found to have Huntington's disease."[15]

Although the L-DOPA load test demonstrated potentially promising results as a possible predictive test for Huntington's disease, it had to be abandoned for several reasons. First, it was impossible to conceal the results of the test because of the nature of the test itself. Some of the people who experienced symptoms similar to those seen in Huntington's disease naturally assumed that the test must be definitive and that, sooner or later, they would get the disease. Even though none of these people were permanently affected by the administration of L-DOPA, some of them became depressed, even suicidal, as a result of their assumption that they had been positively diagnosed with the defective gene. Also, some doctors expressed concern that the test itself might, under certain circumstances, stimulate the biochemical mechanisms involved in the disease and perhaps hasten the onset of symptoms.[16]

For the L-DOPA load test, or any other predictive experiment, to be verified as a reliable procedure, it would have to be repeated many times with uniform success. In this particular case, only ten of thirty persons (33.3 percent) returned a positive result. With such a small sample, this would be quite possible because it *is* a small group and the risk of recurrence for HD declines slowly with advancing age. But, even under ideal conditions, it would take years of further study and watchful waiting to establish the accuracy of this one test. And this leaves still unresolved the ethical and practical problems which forced the experiment to be abandoned.

There are other biochemical approaches to the problem of discovering a presymptomatic detection procedure for Huntington's disease. In 1976 one research team uncovered a promising lead when they found differences in the distribution of gamma-aminobutyric acid (GABA) in the cerebrospinal fluid of persons at risk for the disease. They speculated that these differences could be used to separate the at risk population into two categories—those who carry the gene and those who do not. As in all other forms of predictive research, more detailed study will be necessary to substantiate or disprove this hypothesis. If proven effective, the procedure has the advantages over the L-DOPA load test that prolonged administration of a drug is not necessary, positively tested subjects do not experience symptoms of the disease, and there is no risk of hastening the onset of symptoms. On the other hand, the test requires an invasive technique (lumbar puncture) and measures something that may be a product rather than the root cause of the disease.[17]

Recent advances in technology have been employed in research to develop a presymptomatic detection test for Huntington's disease. One of the most promising of these is computed axial tomographic scanning (popularly known as the "CAT scan"), which is a sophisticated method of x-ray diagnosis of conditions of the brain. An x-ray beam of relatively low dosage is rotated around the head. The x-ray scanning unit takes thousands of rapid readings, which are fed into a computer and processed to yield an actual picture of the brain.[18] If it could be proven that subtle changes in the brain are detectable before symptoms of Huntington's disease become visible, this painless and risk-free procedure might be employed as a predictive test. Unfortunately, preliminary reports on the usefulness of the CAT scan differ. While some research teams are optimistic, others are not. One group in the United States concluded that CAT scanning is useful for confirming a diagnosis of HD, but has no value for predictive purposes at the presymptomatic stage of the disease.[19]

Earlier in this chapter, *genetic linkage studies* were mentioned with reference to the possibility of detecting the HD gene before symptoms appear. These are studies that proceed from the hope that, if the HD gene could be shown to be linked to some other gene, such as that for blood group, its presence and activity could be monitored by following the transmission of the marker gene or genes.[20]

Investigators in various parts of the world are working on this possibility. The task is enormous, somewhat like seeking a needle in a genetic haystack. The possible combinations are so great that many straws will be drawn before the needle is discovered. If a gene *is* found that is closely linked with the gene for HD, then the probability that a particular person at risk carries the HD gene, might be calculated at 5 percent or 95 percent, for example, rather than (as at present) at 50 percent. This result could be refined, perhaps, by assessing other variables such as the subject's age and the onset age of the affected parent, to give even more precise final risk figures. While this would still not represent an unequivocal answer, it would be a great improvement over what is now known. If *two* genetic markers could be located, each with a high probability of linkage with the HD gene, it is conceivable that a definite answer could be given in certain cases. In Melbourne, Australia, David Propert and others who have been working toward this objective have so far excluded about 8 percent of genetic "map units" from serious consideration. Although the road ahead remains long and difficult, genetic linkage analysis holds promise in the struggle to understand and control Huntington's disease.[21]

WHEN SHOULD A PREDICTIVE TEST BE USED?

Some doctors believe that, even if a reliable predictive test for HD is perfected, it should not be made available to the public for general use. They argue that prediction should be held in reserve until the time when the disease can either be cured or managed more effectively. What is the point, they ask, of predicting a condition at a time when medical science can offer only very limited management tools? These doctors are legitimately concerned that the adverse impact of prediction could outweigh any benefits to be gained from it. As one doctor has written,

> The current situation is unhappy enough, but the situation that the invention of such a test will produce may well be worse. At present all offspring of patients with chorea are unhappy at the possibility that they will have [the] disease, but all can also be optimistic that they might escape. The test, however, will divide these offspring into an elated group, who know that they have escaped, and a profoundly unhappy group, who know that they have not. I should like to suggest, therefore, that serious consideration be given to the difficult problems that such a test will bring before, rather than after, its introduction. I should also like to put forward the argument that it is not unreasonable to withhold the use of a test of this sort until we have something tangible to offer to those who give a positive result.[22]

Doctors who disagree with this view maintain that it would be ethically wrong to deny a predictive test to anyone who wished to take it, no matter what the current status of treatment or possible psychological reaction to a positive test. In a free society, people have a right to know that such a test exists, and to make their own informed decision on whether or not to make use of it. If they decide to take the test and then have difficulties adjusting to its result, that is a related but essentially separate issue. These doctors maintain that it is not the role of the researcher to deprive persons of the right to make their own decisions by keeping secret a new predictive test.[23]

Experts who favor the use of a predictive test also emphasize that the test will bring relief and joy to persons who return a negative result. Furthermore, there is always the possibility that more effective treatment, or even a cure, could be discovered between the time the test is taken and the point when symptoms begin to appear. Even if that does not occur, those found to carry the defective gene would be informed about their future. The horrible guessing that is a part of living at risk for the disease would be gone. At the onset of symptoms, those with HD would know what to do and where to turn for help.

Finally, a reliable predictive test would serve as a vital tool for preventive medicine. A person who carries the gene for Huntington's disease will transmit the gene to about half of his or her children. The suffering of those who carry the gene is compounded by the distress and grief of relatives and friends. The cost to society is enormous. The implications for generations yet unborn are incalculable. Use of a predictive test might not save the person tested, but it would at least give him or her more certain grounds on which to consider vasectomy or tubal ligation in order to avoid bringing the same illness upon future generations.

Those at risk for Huntington's disease are well aware of many of these arguments. Long after scientists had begun debating whether or not a presymptomatic detection test for HD should be made available in advance of a cure for the disease, someone finally got around to asking HD families what they thought about the problem. In 1975 Robert Stern and Roswell Eldridge, of the National Institute of Neurological Diseases and Stroke, asked 1,065 HD families in America for their opinion on this matter. Their response indicated that only about 23 percent of persons at risk would refuse a presymptomatic test if it became available.[24]

Since no test is available, where do we stand at the moment? In 1977 the Seventh Workshop on Huntington's disease of the World Federation of Neurology research group on the disorder recommended that "no test should be conducted except for research purposes, and at risk individuals should not be informed of the results since the meaning of the results is still unclear."[25] The debate on the practical and ethical problems associated with the use of a test for the presymptomatic detection of Huntington's disease will continue at least until the time—with luck, in the near future—when a simple, safe, and reliable predictive test is discovered.

7
The Westphal Variant and Juvenile Huntington's Disease

My name is Lynnett. I'm in the fifth grade. My father has had
Huntington's disease all his life that I can remember. We
had to stay by the house to watch him. We had to give medicine
every night. Every year we go around for Huntington's
disease. It can defect the brain. It can make you bad sick, think
wrong, and it makes you mean. You pull off covers and pour
water on people's head. It is a very bad disease. It makes nervous;
you have to leave the house sometime. My mother would get
griped out for being late. He lied on the couch day by day.
One day they might get a cure for it.

Some confusion exists, even within the scientific community, over
the different types of Huntington's disease. Most patients have
the classic choreic type characterized by involuntary muscle
movements, emotional disturbances, and dementia. But a
minority of patients display muscular rigidity rather than chorea.
This type of the disease is called the Westphal variant after
C. F. O. Westphal, who described it in 1883. He mistakenly
believed that it was an entirely new disease, which he called
"pseudosclerosis."[1] The rigid or Westphal variant accounts for
something less than 15 percent of all HD cases. The emotional
and intellectual problems often seen in the choreic form of the
disease are also common in rigid cases.

The existence of a third clinical type, known as the juvenile or
childhood form of the disease, has also been suggested. Onset

in these cases occurs before the age of twenty and may be either choreic or rigid. Not all authorities agree that this is a distinct class of HD; it could be that juvenile cases merely represent "the lower range of the age of onset continuum shown by the former two types." But there do appear to be differences between juvenile-onset and adult-onset cases. Unlike adult-onset HD, the appearance of the disease in children is often accompanied by epilepsy.[2]

Confusion has resulted, not only from uncertainty over whether the juvenile form of the disease represents a distinct clinical type, but also because the term *Westphal variant* has sometimes been used as a synonym for "juvenile Huntington's disease." Children who display symptoms of HD may indeed suffer from the rigid or Westphal type, but this is by no means always the case. Some may even develop it following choreic and convulsive symptoms. The Westphal variant may also be seen in adults. Professor George Bruyn, chairman of the Department of Neurology at University Hospital, Leyden, the Netherlands, has concluded about clinical distinctions between juvenile and adult cases of the Westphal type, "We simply do not know enough about the pathogenetical factors that determine whether a patient will manifest as a juvenile type, a juvenile Westphal type, an adult Westphal type, a type with tardy manifestation, or the usual choreatic type."[3] In this chapter we will examine the general characteristics of the Westphal variant and the peculiarities and problems connected with the onset of HD during childhood.

THE WESTPHAL VARIANT

One of the most significant reasons why the term *Huntington's chorea* has given way to simply *Huntington's disease* is that not all patients with the disorder suffer from involuntary movements. In any group of HD patients, there is considerable variation in both the clinical manifestation of the disease and its natural history or progression. This is true whether the patients have the choreic or the rigid form of the disease. The purpose of classifying a specific variant is to recognize that it does constitute a form of the disease and to try to establish the reasons for the different symptoms which appear.

In an attempt to eliminate some of the confusion that exists regarding the various forms of Huntington's disease, David L. Stevens has proposed the following classification scheme:[4]

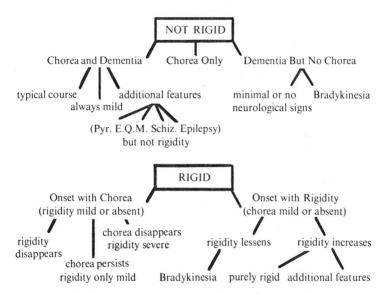

Figure 7.1. Classification scheme for rigid and nonrigid variants of Huntington's disease. From *Advances in Neurology*, edited by A. Barbeau et al. Copyright © 1973 by Raven Press Books, Ltd. Reprinted by permission of Raven Press, New York.

The major division is between the rigid and nonrigid forms of the disease. Stevens has written, "The classification suggested is almost certainly unnecessarily complex and contains too many categories, but, if account had been taken of the wide variety of psychiatric features that can occur, it would be even more complex."[5]

Reporting a typical case of the rigid form of Huntington's disease, M. T. Bird and G. W. Paulson of Ohio State University wrote that their twenty-eight-year-old female patient first noted stiffness of movements at the age of twenty. Daily activities had been well maintained, but had become increasingly difficult. Her eyes tended to lag behind her head movements. She often closed her eyes when turning, her speech was somewhat slurred, and she made occasional "clucking" mouth sounds. Her walking gait was slow and deliberate. She turned her body as a stiff unit. She overbalanced if she tried to turn rapidly.

This woman had the fixed, masklike facial expression which is often characteristic of the rigid form of the disease. Although she read widely, she had difficulty responding to simple questions. The Ohio State doctors reported, "Most of the time she failed to name the President, the governor, or the largest city in the nation. Digit span was only 4 forward, and she could not interpret proverbs."[6]

Although this woman was both physically and intellectually impaired by the disease, it is interesting to note that she was quite self-sufficient in matters of daily living. She could still enjoy doing basic jobs around the house and garden, thereby contributing to the household. Too often in cases just like this, people are sent off to institutions or "homes" where they have little or no opportunity to make use of their remaining skills and abilities.

The woman in this case was relatively young. For reasons we do not understand, rigidity occurs much more often in juvenile cases than in adult patients. The average age of onset for the Westphal variant is thirteen to fourteen years earlier than in choreic cases.[7] Doctors at the University of Wisconsin in Madison reported a typical example of childhood rigidity in a fourteen-year-old girl they called K.C. Patients with the rigid form of HD often come from families with long histories of chorea. This was true of K.C. In juvenile cases, transmission from the father is three or four times as frequent as from the mother. K.C. was typical in this respect, too. Her father, who was first known to have Huntington's disease at the age of twenty-three, died at thirty-eight. Her paternal grandmother and great-grandmother were also known to have had the disease.

K.C. was first admitted to the hospital for evaluation of clumsiness and learning difficulties. As a child her growth and development had been normal, and she was in good health until the age of nine. In the third grade she began to experience difficulty in reading, and her achievement was poor in all subject areas in the fourth grade. Her teachers and parents noted clumsiness, slowness in executing activities, twitching movements in the mouth and face, and slurring of speech. Her face developed a masklike expression, although she smiled readily if coaxed.

The Wisconsin doctors reported that K.C.'s movements were quite distinctive. "The body was moved en bloc; she settled in a chair with a thud and walked stiffly, with no arm swinging and with few other secondary body movements. . . . The patient was unable to move her eyes voluntarily to either the right or the left. . . . Rigidity was readily palpable in all muscle groups but was more marked in the lower extremities." Psychological and intelligence evaluation indicated that K.C. functioned in the moderately retarded range.[8]

In their report, K.C.'s doctors did not specify that she suffered from the Westphal variant of the disease. She displayed both rigidity and some involuntary muscle movement, making specific classification difficult. Reviewing the Anglo-American literature for the period from 1925 to 1968, the doctors found that rigidity was present in 65 percent of the juvenile cases reviewed. It developed early in the course of the disease and was sometimes reported as the first obvious symptom.[9]

Professor Bruyn has noted that rigidity may develop in conjunction with choreic movements, or may emerge as a late or ultimate symptom in the course of the disease. Kenneth Heathfield, of the Regional Centre for Neurology and Neurosurgery in Romford, England, has observed that some patients cease to have chorea and develop a condition resembling Parkinsonism and marked rigidity in the terminal stages of the disease. This terminal rigidity is not an example of the Westphal variant, and should not be confused with it.[10]

Sometimes a fine tremor is an early symptom in cases of the Westphal type. Many patients also develop the posture described by Denny-Brown as typical in cases of damage to a portion of the brain known as the putamen—a raising of the upper arm with a flexed elbow and wrist, and extension of the feet. Epilepsy is common in juvenile HD but conspicuously absent in the Westphal variant. Some of the symptoms that typically differentiate the Westphal variant from the more common choreic variety of HD, Bruyn notes, are impaired ability to perform certain voluntary eye movements and inability to perform various "mimical" tasks, such as "frowning, elevating the eyebrows, blowing-up the cheeks, whistling, showing the teeth, moving about the tongue and protruding it or folding it upon itself." Dementia and impaired speech are frequently associated symptoms. Mutism, emaciation, and skin ulcers may be further complications in advanced cases.[11]

As with the classic form of Huntington's disease, many questions concerning the Westphal variant remain unanswered. What specific mechanism leads to rigidity in this minority of cases? Why is it that rigidity appears to be significantly tied to juvenile onset, yet may develop at any age? What causes the apparently greater loss of specific types of cells in the brain in the Westphal variant? We do not know the answers to these questions. The most likely general explanation is that the Westphal variant is one species of a diversified disorder which is caused by a single, dominant gene but whose various manifestations may be modified by other genes.[12] Colin Brackenridge, formerly of the University of Melbourne, has suggested that some genetic switch, possibly keyed to the age of the affected parent, may be responsible for determining chorea or rigidity, and that this, in turn, influences the age of onset. Thus, patients who develop rigidity are likely to have onset of symptoms at an earlier age than those who develop chorea.[13]

HUNTINGTON'S DISEASE IN CHILDREN

As noted earlier, the experts disagree as to whether Huntington's disease in children is a distinct clinical variant. The Westphal variant is considered a separate entity because it has different characteristics from those of the classic form of the disease. Bruyn wrote in 1968 that the juvenile type of Huntington's disease "does possess a character all its own and, from the clinical point of view, is justifiably recognized as a particular type or phenotypic variant of the disease." But Bruyn also noted that it is pointless to argue over the true age of onset of a genetic disorder which, strictly speaking, is present from the moment of conception.[14] Many experts would argue that childhood HD is simply an overt appearance of the disease at an earlier time in life than that at which it is normally seen.

Specialists who have studied juvenile-onset Huntington's disease have established that patients with onset of symptoms before the age of twenty compose between 5 and 10 percent of all cases of the disease. Onset is frequently of the rigid form, and epileptic seizures are present in about half these patients. The duration of the disease is usually shorter than in adult-onset cases. Death occurs after an average of about eight years. The symptoms often progress more rapidly and are more severe than in Huntington's disease of late onset.[15]

Studying data collected on 150 juvenile cases of the disease, Bruyn observed that definitive diagnosis is nearly impossible if the presence of hereditary chorea cannot be confirmed in the family's history.[16] Other investigators have pointed out that many cases are misdiagnosed, often as Wilson's disease and post-encephalitic Parkinsonism.[17] The diagnostic problem is frequently complicated by the presence of epilepsy, which is more common in childhood-onset than in adult-onset HD, and by mental retardation, which often makes swift progress in childhood-onset HD.[18]

When HD appears in children, it usually does so during the second decade of life. Appearance of the disease during the first decade is rare but not unknown. In 1967, one medical team reported details of the disease in four children in whom the onset of symptoms came before age ten. In three of the four patients, symptoms appeared before the age of five. This is very unusual, but a summary of one of these cases will usefully illustrate some of the clinical and social problems presented by HD of very early onset.[19]

Linda was admitted to the Children's Hospital Medical Center in Boston after "complaints of progressively clumsy rigid gait, leaning forward while walking, speech impairment, weakness, and loss of appetite, all commencing between $4\frac{1}{2}$ and 5 years of age." Upon being interviewed, Linda's mother said that there was no hint of neurological disease in the family. Although Linda had difficulty walking and speaking, psychological testing indicated mental capabilities that were about right for her age.

For the next two years Linda visited a chiropractor. Her condition did not improve, and she returned to the hospital for further tests shortly before her eighth birthday. By this time, she dragged her left leg and held her left arm stiffly at her side when walking. She sometimes lost consciousness and collapsed backwards. Coordination of hands and feet was unsatisfactory. Her school performance had been so poor that she was repeating the first grade. Her speech had improved somewhat, but it was still indistinct and immature. She burst into laughter at odd times, and often grimaced. She was unable to stand on one leg without falling. Her gait was rigid and shambling, with a tendency to walk on the left toes. Blood, urine, and other standard laboratory tests showed results that were generally within the normal range. However, a photograph of the brain indicated abnormalities in the lateral ventricles and other problems that are often specifically associated with Huntington's disease and similar disorders.

Regular checks were made on Linda over the next four years. By the time she had reached the age of eight years and eight months, involuntary grimacing of the type often seen in adult HD was clearly evident. Myoclonic seizures became so frequent that Linda had to wear a hockey helmet during most of her waking hours to minimize the danger of injury. By this time she had been removed from school.

At the age of eleven, Linda's speech was almost incomprehensible. Her emotions were volatile, and she suffered periodically from grand mal convulsions. Unable to swallow hard food, she subsisted almost entirely on milk, ice cream, juices, and jellies. She could not walk, except on her knees. Six months later she was bedridden and very rigid. She could still gesture with her right hand, and seemed to recognize her parents and her doctor, but could no longer speak. Treatment with a variety of drugs was mostly unsuccessful in relieving her suffering.

After Linda had been under observation for some time, her five-year-old brother was brought to the medical center because he had symptoms like his sister's. His mother continued to deny the presence of any neurological problem in the family. With *both* children in the hospital, their father finally came to visit them for the first time. The doctors later recorded their reaction. "When he walked into the ward, it was apparent that he had a somewhat rigid gait, that he grimaced frequently, and that his hands were unsteady with occasional twitching movements. He consented to attempt a drawing of a tree which consisted of an ill-formed circle on top of a single line—a very primitive representation. Thereafter, he refused to submit to further examination or discuss his children's disease." His wife then confessed that she had denied the presence of illness in the family because her husband had ordered her to do so. She also admitted that during the past few years he had become progressively withdrawn and emotionally unstable. He wrecked the car several times. His skills in an automobile assembly plant had deteriorated to the point that he was relegated to a simpler job, with a loss in pay. He had become restless and unhappy. Friends took him for drunk when he had not taken a single drink. He was only thirty-one years old.

The family history revealed that this man's father had died in a mental hospital at the age of forty-four. He had been diagnosed with Huntington's disease. Relatives testified that the presence of the disease could be traced for at least three generations, but the family had become skilled at denying and concealing it.[20]*

Linda's case illustrates another puzzling aspect of Huntington's disease in children. As previously noted, the disease is most often inherited from the father.[21] This pattern does not appear to be simply a reflection of the relative fertility of the parents, because the fertility of affected females is thought to be greater than that of affected males at all ages of onset.[22] A different hypothesis focuses on maternal-fetal interaction. The idea is that the HD gene is active in some cases even during the fetal stage of development, and that a fetus with both the HD gene and a predisposition to childhood onset succumbs in the womb if the mother also carries the gene.[23] There is little evidence at present to support this theory.

A related but more complex hypothesis holds that there are early-onset modifier genes which are somehow sex-linked. It is theorized that these modifiers, when present in the mother, could

---

* J. E. Oliver and K. E. Dewhurst have suggested that because families are so skilled at concealing the disease, especially when it strikes children, the incidence of childhood and adolescent forms of HD may be higher than commonly believed.

act upon the HD gene in such a way as to discriminate against the production of affected offspring and in favor of the birth of unaffected children.[24]

There are many other theories involving possible sex-related factors in the inheritance of juvenile Huntington's disease.[25] Colin Brackenridge and Betty Teltscher have suggested that age of onset is related both to the age of onset in the affected parent and to the age of the affected parent when a child is born. Certainly it is clear, as Brackenridge and others have shown, that early onset, rigidity, and high frequency of affected fathers are closely associated factors.[26]

For years, there has been speculation that hereditary diseases tend to show earlier onset and more pronounced symptoms with each passing generation. It is thought by some that more juvenile cases are appearing because of this. This postulated phenomenon is sometimes called "anticipation." There has been considerable debate as to whether anticipation is a clinical fact or the product of earlier and better diagnosis of the disease. Some experts believe that the debate is impossible to resolve "because of the chronological difficulties of the same observer undertaking a detailed study of the development of the disease through three or more generations." It is probable that anticipation is influenced to a significant extent by "the artifact of more diligent observation."[27] The disease is detected earlier, or concealed less, with each passing generation. This is particularly true in recent times, because some of the stigma associated with hereditary disease has been lifted, and public attitudes have improved. The skills and interest of the scientific community have also been sharpened.

Social and Psychological Problems
Associated with Huntington's Disease in Children

Children with Huntington's disease must often contend both with a particularly virulent form of the disorder and with a whole range of associated social and psychological problems. Some of these problems may be present before a child shows any symptom of the disease. They may continue even if a child who is at risk does not have the disorder. For example, in one study of 172 at risk children, twelve were illegitimate, seventeen were seriously neglected, and nine had been subjected to acts of extreme violence.[28]

In a study of the social and psychological impact of Huntington's disease in Northamptonshire, England, Jack E. Oliver documented cases of neglect, assault, illegitimacy, abandonment, alcoholism, criminality, death by accident, and one case in which a child had been murdered.[29] A young Australian woman told David C. Wallace how she let her Huntingtonian father drive off a pier into Townsville harbor in a rainstorm while she sat passively beside him because she was frightened by his anger when his least whim was crossed. Her father drowned, and she narrowly escaped with her life.[30]

Dr. Wallace observed that the disease can have a devastating impact on some families, especially the children.

> The household in which they grow up is frequently grossly disturbed. A father becoming demented [is] restless, moving from job to job, always in a downward direction, dragging his hapless family with him, unkind to his wife and frequently brutal to his children. A woman becoming demented will sit watching television all day while the flies crawl over the breakfast laid out on the table among the remains of the meal from the night before . . . careless of the welfare of her husband and children. The husband then frequently takes to alcohol and the children to juvenile delinquency. Or sometimes worse than this, the husband will leave home. . . .
>
> Yet there is no way in which one can be sure who will be affected and who will not [among the children]. The household is frequently so disturbed that no normal child could grow up in it psychologically unscathed, so all the children may have some psychological abnormalities.[31]

Even the trained observer coming into contact with such a family might conclude that a child at risk was showing early signs of HD when the child was free of the gene but psychologically disturbed by a chaotic home environment. A child who did carry the gene and had begun to show early symptoms of the disease would be required to cope with the onset of the disease *and* the impossible domestic situation as well. Since children are less able to protect themselves than adults, and defenseless against capricious actions, the consequences can be unbelievably tragic.

The five thick volumes of public testimony collected by the U.S. Commission for the Control of Huntington's Disease and Its Consequences are replete with personal histories of many hundreds of people who have experienced some of these problems. A summary of the experiences of one family provides an illustration. This is not an extreme example. There are more horrific cases on record.

In 1952, Mrs. Don Jones of Big Spring, Texas, noticed that her young husband was growing more and more irritable. He became very nervous and rather awkward. Within a few years he lost several jobs, and Mrs. Jones had to go to work. By that time, the couple had two children. In 1957 Don's condition became so serious that he sought help at a local hospital. He was diagnosed as having a "nervous condition" and given electric shock treatments. His symptoms only got worse. He returned home, no longer able to hold a job, and did not visit the hospital again until 1960. On that occasion he was examined by a panel of doctors, who diagnosed Huntington's disease. An investigation into the family history revealed that Don's father had been diagnosed in a Kansas hospital as suffering from "postinfluenzal encephalitis." The Big Spring panel concluded that this had been a misdiagnosis and the family carried the gene for Huntington's disease.

In 1962 Don was readmitted to the hospital for custodial care. For five years the family had subsisted on his wife's meager income and modest Social Security payments. Don was not a veteran and therefore not eligible for ex-servicemen's benefits.

By the time Don was actually diagnosed in 1960 (at least eight years after onset), his ten-year-old son, Stephen, had already begun manifesting symptoms of the disease. The boy had been a superior student until he reached the fourth grade. Then he began to fall behind. Writing became more difficult for him, and he feigned illness to get out of school. Finally, Stephen was taken to the hospital for tests. They revealed nothing abnormal.

By mid-1964, Don had weakened so much that all his food had to be blended to prevent him from choking. By Thanksgiving in November, he could no longer swallow at all. He died in January, 1965, from the effects of starvation and a weakened heart.

Stephen was now fifteen years old, and his condition had also deteriorated. He stumbled, had "blackout spells," and often fell as a result. His classmates at school called him "a mental case." They teased and attacked him unmercifully. His younger sister, also at risk for HD, was heartbroken in her vain attempts to protect him. The family's pediatrician, who now knew that the family carried the gene for HD, told them that Huntington's chorea only appeared in males.

In October, 1966, Stephen had his first grand mal seizure. The pediatrician confirmed epilepsy but dismissed the possibility of Huntington's disease on the theory that the boy was too young. Medications were prescribed, but the seizures grew more frequent. Early in 1967, Stephen visited a neurologist in Lubbock, Texas, and a diagnosis of HD was confirmed. The family returned home in despair. A year later Stephen fell and injured an ankle. Except for a brief period, he never walked again. Gradually, he became a complete invalid. During the last year of his life, he was totally dependent on others. His mother testified about those final months,

> He was not able to hold up his head; sometimes the frustrations would bring on petit mal (sometimes, grand mal) seizures, making it more difficult to feed him. He went through repetitious pneumonia, several hospitalizations; and the last was a cruel 39 days. . . . He had trouble with collapsing veins, retention of some 30 or 40 pounds of fluid from the I.V.'s. His skin was stretched almost to bursting. . . . Finally, pneumonia, a weakened heart and a merciful God allowed him to pass from his torment. [He] was only 19 years old. . . . [32]

Coping with Huntington's Disease in Children

Most of the management tools discussed in chapter 5 of this book apply equally to adult and childhood forms of Huntington's disease. Some suggestions for young people are also given in chapter 8. Several additional observations may prove useful to some families in which Huntington's disease is present.

When HD appears in a loved one, especially a child, it is easy for other members of the family to become too protective. In his excellent book, *Living With Chronic Neurologic Disease*, I. S. Cooper has warned, "It is generally not necessary for a partially disabled person to become totally parasitic or for a devoted parent to become totally servile. It is not good for the patient and not good for the family. Be aware of this danger. Avoid it as gracefully and intelligently as possible."[33] If the family becomes excessively protective, everyone may gradually become "locked into the patient's illness and the secondary emotional consequences":

> Some children, as well as certain aging parents and disabled husbands and wives, come to use their dependent situation to control the family. This may not be conscious behavior on the part of the patient, although, surprisingly enough, many patients have actually admitted that they are using their disability to manipulate those about them.
>
> If you become totally permissive, totally giving, then the patient, like a spoiled child, may become tyrannical in his demands for attention. Even when all members of a family are in relatively good health, it is not uncommon to find that one person, seemingly less independent than the others, psychologically controls the family situation. Achieving the delicate balance in which each child receives the attention he needs, while none is allowed to dominate, is certainly one of the major tasks which must be accomplished when raising children. The situation in caring for chronically ill individuals is not dissimilar.[34]

Management of any chronic disease in childhood should be directed toward minimizing the damaging consequences of the disease while "maximizing a mature acceptance of the child's real strengths and realistic limitations." The damaging consequences of the disease may involve not only the affected child, but other members of the family as well, especially the mother. When childhood illness contributes to an anxiety-dominated relationship between mother and child, it "virtually ensures that neither party will be able to handle the disease and its consequences without substantial neurotic overlay."[35]

It is also important for parents to remember that children often interpret life and their own experiences quite differently from adults. In Australia, Professor David Maddison and Beverley Raphael have pointed out some aspects of child development which are relevant for parents of children who are troubled by chronic disease. For example, the feelings of a seriously ill child under the age of five years are frequently determined by the threat of separation from its parents (as in hospitalization). When the child is between five and ten years of age, the major fear may be of mutilation which the youngster thinks may result from some form of treatment. Concern for one's own mortality, a fear of death, usually emerges as the chief concern "only after the age of ten years."[36]

Passivity and feelings of helplessness, inadequacy, or guilt may be present in children even before the age of ten. As the child moves into adolescence, these feelings may combine with isolation and a variety of other problems to seriously undermine the ability to establish any clear concept of role or identity. If the young person has early-onset HD, with progressive dementia, emotional instability, and chorea, any satisfactory role identification may be almost impossible to achieve.

Day-by-day coping with Huntington's disease in children is largely a matter of good common sense. Provide the child with reassurance, love, and help without encouraging dependency. Give the child the maximum scope for self-expression and activity without allowing him, or the illness, to dominate the household. All the lessons of adult management are applicable: plan the day, incorporate a reasonable variety of activities, encourage exercise, develop hobbies, encourage the child not to retreat or give up any social function he can manage, and don't worry too much about what the public may think. Other members of the family should find someone to talk to about *their* problems. Assure "islands of fun and pleasure" for the patient and for everyone in the family each day. Other members of the family must have time of their own, a period every day when they are freed from the responsibility of caring for someone.[37]

Cooper has written, "*Coping with the daily burdens of caring for someone who is chronically ill is itself a form of chronic illness. . . .* The families of the chronically ill have generally been as desperately in need of help as the patients." When families understand that stress is natural and take steps to cope with it, they usually find that the home atmosphere improves markedly. Even if the disease is progressive, it need not be allowed to drag otherwise healthy people in its wake. When persons responsible for a chronically ill relative provide for independent time and "avoid or clean out the anger, resentment and guilt that beleaguer so many," they avoid the traps of self-pity and martyrdom, and are able to enjoy life fully.[38]

When it becomes clear that the patient will never fully regain his health, some very difficult questions inevitably arise. Dr. Cooper reminds us that when we get depressed and ask, "Is it really worth all of this effort?" the answer should come ringing back, "Yes, it is worth the effort. People are, essentially, for each other: to be good companions, to be active, to try to keep their own health, and to help persons dear to them to regain theirs. There are no viable alternatives."[39] When the disease is progressive and full recovery impossible, it is vital that the family work together to assure that everyone enjoys the fullest life possible.

8
Social Problems

*The one thing that impresses me most about the disease . . . is
that it's so debilitating, not only physically, but socially.
People just don't understand what it is, and you become sort
of an outcast from society. People stare at you, and they
don't understand what's wrong. Even when they do know
what disease it is, it's sort of like you have the plague,
or something.*

The number of people who are actually affected by Huntington's
disease is relatively small, but the impact of the disorder on
society as a whole is enormous. The burden falls, not just on the
person who has the disease, but upon the children who are at risk
for it, and upon the spouse, relatives, friends, neighbors, employers, the medical profession, and various authorities. In economic
terms, the cost runs to many millions of dollars.

When viewed in this light, it is clear that the incidence figures for
Huntington's disease—six or seven per hundred thousand—if
taken at face value, are misleading.[1] Medical files are filled with
statistics, testimonials, case studies, and letters bearing witness to
the widespread psychological and social trauma caused by HD
and related disorders. Consider, for example, the following letter
selected at random from hundreds which were addressed to the
U. S. Commission for the Control of Huntington's Disease. The
writer, who is from Arizona, asked to remain anonymous:

15 April 1977
My beloved husband died of Huntington's disease at the age

of 39 years. We had married in 1919 when I was 17 and he was 18. He was a handsome youth. We lived with his parents at the beginning of our marriage, and his mother was afflicted with the disease at that time. She died in 1927. His grandmother and an aunt died from Huntington's, and an uncle committed suicide when he learned he had the disease.

At this time we did not even know what the ailment was called and no treatment was given. The unfortunate victims were hidden most of the time. It was considered a disgrace to mention their problem. Many times they were mistaken for drunk and arrested if alone on the street.

My handsome husband and I had a happy life for four years. During that time we were blessed with a son, a beautiful baby who died at the age of three. Then we were advised by a doctor to have no more children. This made the baby's death more tragic than ever. My husband never fully recovered from the shock of the baby's death. Shortly after this, he showed signs of nervousness, and I've often wondered if this bereavement hastened the progress of the disease.

He would never admit he was afflicted, although the disease progressed rapidly. He lost his good looks, could not hold a job, and was accused of drunkenness many times. So he took to drink. He was very popular in his youth, admired by both men and women, and a friend to all; but they deserted him when he needed them the most.

Finally he was placed in a mental institution. When the orderlies came to take him away, he resisted with all his feeble strength and cried out to me to help him. I will never forget this dreadful event. I tried to take care of him until he became dangerous to himself and others before I made this dreadful decision; and to this day, I regret it. He refused to eat, and beer was all he wanted. He died of starvation after 18 months in the mental institution. God bless his soul. . . .[2]

This anguished account touches on some of the many social problems associated with Huntington's disease—public ignorance, stigmatization, desertion by friends, problems with employers and the authorities, real and imagined drunkenness, concealment of the disease, institutionalization, suicide. The list could be extended almost indefinitely with stories like this one. The presence of the disease, or even the threat of it, can disrupt engagements, marriages, and family life. To make a bad situation much worse, the financial burden imposed by the disease may force the family over the brink of poverty. The physical, emotional, and economic toll can overpower and ruin many lives.

Perhaps the least necessary of the many forms of unhappiness experienced by families with Huntington's disease is that caused by public insensitivity. Hundreds of examples could be cited to illustrate the damage caused when people act with medieval ignorance. We will examine only one, of a man moderately disabled by HD who was institutionalized for threatening neighborhood children. On one occasion he chased a group of children down the street and kicked at the front door when they retreated into a house. Complaints were filed, and the man was ordered into a psychiatric hospital. Later investigation proved that his actions were prompted not so much by the presence of the disease as by the children themselves, who tormented and teased him because they thought he was "a crazy man." They mocked him and threw stones and garbage whenever he appeared outside his house. They made games of luring him into traps where he tripped over a hidden wire or fell into some ambush. When he finally struck back, the parents of the children phoned the police and demanded that this "dangerous man be put away for good." One neighbor even complained that having a man on the block who was "a mental case" tended to "lower the moral tone and the property values in the whole area."

Clearly, even in the most enlightened times, the mean and hurtful actions of a few people can make public places frightening for the innocently afflicted. Social smashups that occur when HD is present are rarely the patient's fault; a great many "normal" people contribute to ruinous incidents by their ignorance, insensitivity, or selfishness.

When disease, ignorance, and lack of compassion are all intertwined, though, it is perhaps pointless to talk about who is at "fault." Usually placing blame doesn't really help much. The case studies cited in this book have revealed suffering so deep that it strains the expressive limits of language. That suffering is what we should keep always in mind, with the steady object of finding and eliminating its causes, rather than unprofitably fixing blame on this person or that.

Overcoming public ignorance is not always sufficient. In the case described above, some of the neighborhood children threw stones even after they were told that the man suffered from a serious illness and could not help the way he walked. Their parents, who did not throw stones, persisted in their attempts to have the man permanently removed from the community. Possibly the International Year for Disabled Persons, inaugurated by the United Nations for 1981, will accelerate the movement to achieve overdue reforms and improved public attitudes, especially toward the mentally handicapped.

FAMILY PROBLEMS

Sometimes the social consequences of Huntington's disease seem more intractable than the illness itself. This is particularly true within the family, where the first social impact is usually experienced. Some family problems were discussed in chapter 7, but there are many others. Consider another brief case study.

Mrs. C. Ramsay began to show symptoms of Huntington's disease at the age of thirty-five. Her choreic movements gradually became more severe. Her husband and two teenaged children were not troubled by her physical disability as much as by her irritability and pathological jealousy, particularly toward her husband. She demonstrated no severe memory deterioration, but became careless and unclean. The family tried to conceal her illness from friends. When this was no longer possible, they isolated themselves. This was not difficult, because former friends gradually drifted away.

Mr. Ramsay soon found himself in a difficult dilemma. His wife had become unpredictable and unattractive, yet extremely jealous. He remained faithful and devoted to her but could no longer bring himself to have sexual relations with her. Her sex life ceased entirely, and Mr. Ramsay eventually had an affair with another woman. He now felt guilty because he believed he had finally committed the sin of which his wife had accused him for many years.[3]

How is a family to cope with problems like these? What advice is to be given? Is Mr. Ramsay morally obligated to remain sexually faithful to his wife, or is his real problem not so much what he did as the guilt he feels for having done it? In situations of this type there are no perfect answers. Unfortunately, this does not prevent some people from giving "definitive" advice. Chapter 4 in this book began with a quotation from a woman whose parents sought a birth control dispensation from the parish priest because the mother had Huntington's disease. The priest told them that there were no exceptions. Rather than take or use contraceptives, the couple did not have intercourse.[4]

Families who face problems similar to that of the Ramsays must work out their own solutions, taking into account their unique circumstances and ethical convictions. They should be aware that social pressures can unduly influence their decisions. In many localities, for example, it would be considered socially tolerable for Mr. Ramsay to seek sexual fulfillment outside his marriage, but intolerable for Mrs. Ramsay to do the same if she happened to be the healthy partner. Individual or family decisions on matters of vital personal significance should be guided more by genuinely believed ethical considerations than by prevailing social norms, which may be distinctly unfair.

Nor can the family afford to ignore the personal needs of the person who has the disease. Consideration in the above discussion is given to the sexual dilemma of the healthy spouse. What about the partner who is ill? Mrs. Ramsay's neurological disorder does not necessarily end her sexual desire or dictate that it must be starved. Dr. I. S. Cooper has noted that, in recent years, something of a "sexual revolution of the neurologically handicapped has begun." We can no longer ignore or deny "that erotic element which is imprisoned within a contorted body. . . . "[5] Because Huntington's disease is a neurological disorder which is also *hereditary*, of course, great care must be taken that sexual activity does not lead inadvertently to procreation. But the way in which many people would resolve this problem, by insisting that everyone with HD abstain from any form of sexual expression, is both unfair and unrealistic. In some situations, advice about masturbation may be precisely what is most needed to help a neurologically handicapped person. Naturally, if everyone else is too embarrassed or too biased even to consider the subject, it is not likely that the handicapped person will receive such advice. Old prejudices must be conquered. Fixed ideas must be made more flexible. On these matters of great personal importance, people need to talk to each other openly and frankly.

For some couples, sexual compatibility is not a significant problem by the time Huntington's disease appears. For others, it is an aspect of life which should not be ignored. Dr. Cooper recommends specialized sexual counseling in such cases. He advises, "Don't allow your neurologically disabled child or spouse to become a sexual neuter. Learn to break down your own hang-ups, so that you can understand the disabled person's problems about sexual attitudes and behavior."[6]

Many problems in the everyday household management of Huntington's disease can be avoided by making relatively minor adjustments. Converting to unbreakable dishes or a serving cart rather than a tray, for example, can help preserve the HD patient's ability to contribute to household welfare.

After-dinner activities should not be forgotten. Many moderately impaired HD patients enjoy a simple game of cards with the family. Checkers are sometimes possible, especially if a large board and big, stable pieces are provided. In more serious cases, the patient may be able to act as "advisor" to someone directly involved in the game. There are many simple, safe games and activities which can be used to brighten the day for the whole family. Experiment. Explore possibilities. Look for ideas and activities that the HD member of the family may find interesting or enjoyable. An evening at a concert (especially an outdoor concert), a visit to a close friend, a trip to a ball game, a walk in the park—all these activities, alternating with quieter evenings spent with television or recorded music, add interest to life. If there is a musician in the family, HD patients will often be cheered by a sing-along. Cultivating activities that involve the person who has the disease may require some thought and work, but the rewards are worth the effort.

Beware of the tendency to exclude an affected person from the conversation without realizing it. A woman in Los Angeles whose mother had Huntington's disease observed, "A lot of people talk about my mother and not [to] her. I know I did it for a long time myself and sometimes catch myself doing it. The person with HD is sort of regarded as not there."[7] Many patients in the advanced stages of the disease are still able to comprehend most of what goes on around them. They may respond in a limited way, but that does not mean they should be ignored. Try not to talk about them. Talk *to* them.

It is often easier to talk to someone you haven't seen for a few days or weeks. The task of caring for an HD patient *all* the time can be too demanding. Everyone needs a break now and then. Many Huntington's disease associations around the world now participate in respite care programs whereby the patient can "take a holiday" away from the family. This may be either at a care center in the same city or at a resort location some distance away. With provision for proper care, families can also make private holiday arrangements. However it is done, regular holiday breaks benefit both the patient and the rest of the family.

YOUNG PEOPLE

Not enough has been written about the impact of Huntington's disease on young people in the family. In the previous chapter, some attention was given to the problems that arise when the disease actually strikes a young person. This happens only in a small minority of cases, because HD usually appears much later in life. Nevertheless, in families where the gene for the disorder is known to be present, young people may face a triple challenge. While facing the usual uncertainties of adolescence, they may be trying to come to terms with their own risk for HD and contributing to the care of a patient who has the disease. At a time when most of their peers have no greater responsibility than doing school work and carrying out the garbage, they may face responsibilities which would test the courage and will of the most mature adult. Their social life may be disrupted, their free time limited, and it may even be necessary for them to contribute something to the family income.

In some extreme cases, the children in the family may be subjected to the threat of violence. One woman in a small town in Kansas broke into tears when she spoke of the behavior of her husband, who had Huntington's disease: "Whenever he was feeling good . . . he was kind. And then, there would be times that he was so vicious and mean that you wouldn't realize just exactly how mean that a person could get to his own loved ones. He'd beat me, he'd beat the children, he'd break things. It was just like a completely different person than what we were used to."[8]

A twenty-year-old man from the same state reported a similar experience.

> My mother developed this fear that someone would see her in her deteriorating condition, so I lived for years in a house that was continually dark. Every window was covered by venetian blinds or shades, or even pieces of cardboard. . . .
>
> One of my most prevalent memories was that she always stood in the corner of the kitchen gazing at nothing and smoking an endless stream of cigarettes. The few attempts I made in communicating with her were usually spent in trying to make her smile, or at least respond. She was so moody and silent and I just wanted her to know that I cared. I never remember her touching or kissing me, which in a way reflects the isolation and distance that was felt throughout our family.
>
> Some other memories concern my family, such as losing her temper. She usually did this with the second oldest child. Sometimes she'd whip him until a yardstick would break and she'd continue doing it, and end up stabbing him several times.[9]

Obviously, this is the kind of family situation that must be avoided. The mother is isolated, inactive, depressed, and sometimes violent. During her periods of violence, the life of one of her children is endangered. Are young people helpless in a home environment like this? What is to be done?

Young readers of this book who have parents with HD should take courage from knowing that they are not alone. No one has been singled out to serve lonely duty in "the school of hard knocks." There are other young people in the locality, in the nation, and throughout the world who face similar problems. All share the common experience of living in a family where a serious hereditary disorder is present. When the U.S. Commission for the Control of Huntington's Disease toured the country, accepting public testimony about the disorder, hundreds of young people came forward to share their experiences or to plead for assistance for friends in an HD family. You may find it useful to contact some of these people, either through your local HD chapter or through some similar organization. Sharing your problems is a good first step toward overcoming them.

You may also find it helpful to find a wise and compassionate friend to whom you can turn for advice. It may be a relative, a neighbor, someone at church, a doctor, or a school counselor. The person should be old enough and mature enough to understand your problems and offer advice if you need help. This is particularly important if there is violence at home.

Living with a relative who has Huntington's disease may call for considerable sacrifice on your part, but it does not mean that you must endure physical abuse. In a minority of HD families, the domestic situation can become dangerous, particularly to young people, who are not always in a position to protect themselves. Modern drugs are usually adequate to prevent HD patients who require special treatment from becoming dangerous to themselves or to other members of the family. But this is not always the case, and sometimes drugs are not available or may not be taken.

If a family member with HD is known to have bouts of unpredictable or violent behavior, proper steps must be taken to protect all concerned, including the person who has the disease. Some families continue to live with the threat of violence month after month and year after year as if there were nothing to be done about it. That is no way to live. It is not normal or necessary for any household to be subjected to random terror, whether the problem is Huntington's disease or something else (alcoholism, for example, which sometimes compounds the task of managing Huntington's disease).

Any young person who is subjected to the threat of violence should be able to seek protection. This is one reason why it is important to have a mature person at hand who can assist in times of crisis. In most localities there are also constituted authorities who are charged with the responsibility of intervening in just such crises. It may be the police, child welfare authorities, a social worker, or a member of the clergy. Whoever the responsible people are, the important thing is to get in touch with them and seek help.

For most young people in HD families, the threat of violence is not present. The real difficulty is living in a household where illness is always present. Over the long haul, this can become very demoralizing. Young people should try to remember that their job is to contribute to the remedy, not to the problem. Carry your fair share of the load, but be honest and gentle with yourself as well as with others. Try not to be overly sensitive to public attitudes and reactions. What people do not understand often frightens them. That is why people stare when you are out in public with an HD relative or friend. If you sometimes feel that life is unfair, and you find yourself asking, "Why me?" consider that there is much to be learned, even from adversity. Do not allow the adversity to blind you to the simple and enjoyable things in life. Strive to be happy.

OTHER SOCIAL PROBLEMS

While it is impossible to discuss in detail all the social problems that may arise as a result of Huntington's disease, a few examples may prove illuminating.

One of the most common complaints among HD families is that the person with the disease has been mistakenly arrested for drunkenness. The characteristic unsteady walk of the HD patient can easily mislead the police. Sometimes an arrest is followed by a traumatic and unnecessary night in jail. Relatives are justifiably upset when an innocent person is thus subjected to a painful and humiliating experience.

Educating the police is not the answer. Even if the police were made aware of the disorder, it would be unfair to expect a patrolman to make a medical diagnosis on a darkened street. A better approach is to provide the patient with identification which describes the disease and names a reliable contact in the event of trouble. There are a number of ways to do this. A card containing the information can be placed in a wallet or purse. In most countries, "Medic Alert" bracelets are available. It is also possible to sew a small patch onto the clothing.

Some social problems associated with Huntington's disease are clearly the responsibility of the patient and the family. For example, many people who are diagnosed with the disease continue to drive an automobile long after it is safe for them to do so. Men, in particular, seem to derive much self-esteem from driving. To abandon driving is to admit that their functional abilities are declining. But to continue driving is to endanger themselves, their loved ones, and other members of the community. The family may have to exercise firm pressure to assure that the HD patient gives up the privilege of driving in good time.

Another common problem among HD families is the fear of discrimination in employment. One of the chief reasons Huntingtonian families still attempt to hide the disease is the fear that their livelihood will be endangered if an employer discovers that a serious, hereditary disorder exists in the family. Voluntary organizations to combat HD have difficulty attracting young members, partly because some young people fear that membership could jeopardize their career opportunities. The employer could find out about the disease and conclude that the employee is a poor long-term career risk. Some people who are not even endangered by the disease may give HD groups a wide berth for the same reason.

The undeniable discrimination that prompts these fears is unforgivable. In some countries, it is also illegal. Employers may be in violation of the law if they discriminate against a disabled person or anyone who is at risk for a disabling disease. In the United States, all departments of the federal government are prohibited from discriminating against handicapped persons. They are also required to submit to the U.S. Civil Service Commission "affirmative action" plans for the hiring, placement, and advancement of disabled employees.

Persons who do not work for federal agencies or federal contractors in the United States may not enjoy the protection of similar legislation. State laws vary greatly on these matters, as does legislation from one country to the next. These disparities make it essential that groups concerned about equality of treatment should insist upon protective legislation everywhere which is backed by sufficient enforcement procedures to make it effective.[10]

Ironically, some HD families discriminate against themselves. They do so by failing to take advantage of services which have been designed for their use. This may happen because the family does not know the services are available. Sometimes it happens because the family is "too proud" to accept assistance. There is nothing wrong with being proud at the proper time, but pride should not come before good sense. A father who is too proud to seek or accept community aid is not to be excused if his family suffers. Many HD families have legitimate needs. In most countries, the government and various public agencies have attempted to provide for some of those needs. Some countries have done better than others in this regard. But if a family ignores available services, the best program in the world is useless.

When HD families do seek advice, they often ask about adoption. This is particularly true of young, married couples who are considering the alternative of adoption because one partner is at risk for the disease. Laws governing adoption vary so widely that only a few general observations are appropriate here. Your local authorities or HD group should be able to offer more specific information applicable to where you live.

In some localities a decree of adoption will not be granted to a couple in whom the risk for HD is present, because the courts have concluded that the potential burden of the disease is so serious that placement in such a home would not be in the best long-term interests of the child. For this reason, some couples who are eager to adopt a child may not mention the disease. This is unwise. Couples have a moral obligation, and usually a legal duty as well, to tell the whole truth. Concealing important information which may have a bearing on the life of another person is not an acceptable practice no matter how desperately the couple may wish to adopt a child.

Couples who are not eligible to adopt, or who are denied a decree of adoption, may feel that they have been mistreated. They should try to keep in mind that the most common criterion for adoption is "the best interests of the child." If placement of a child in a specific family is not deemed to be in that child's best interests, the courts may deny the placement "no matter how unfair or cruel the decision may appear when viewed from the perspective of the prospective adoptive parents."[11] Realizing this may be small comfort to the couple that has just been denied a decree of adoption, but it is something that should be clearly understood.

In some localities, being at risk for HD is not a bar to successful adoption. Many couples with one spouse at risk for the disease have adopted a child quite successfully. Some who have faced long waiting lists have improved their chances by showing interest in a child who is considered difficult to place. This may include handicapped children or, in some cases, babies of mixed race. Under these special circumstances, it may be that the best interests of the child *are* served by adoption by a person who is at risk for Huntington's disease.[12]

If adoption is impossible, there are other alternatives which should be considered. One solution may be to act as very involved godparents in something akin to an extended family situation. Nieces and nephews are usually very receptive to the special attention and care offered by affectionate godparents.

Medical research has rapidly advanced another alternative which might be called a "genetic bypass." For couples in whom the male is at risk for the disease, artificial insemination using a sperm donor (A.I.D.) may be a possibility. By this means the parents can have a baby after a normal pregnancy, with no chance that the father's genetic risk will be inherited by the child. Unfortunately, there is at present no comparable procedure for cases in which the woman is the one at risk.[13]

CONCLUSION

A discussion of the social implications of Huntington's disease could be extended almost indefinitely. Problems related to guardianship, conservatorship, hospital and nursing home admissions, involuntary commitment, confidentiality, probate, and so on all deserve detailed discussion, but local regulations vary so greatly that it is impossible to address these problems in a book intended for general use.[14]

We have seen how the "ripple effect" which occurs when Huntington's disease is present can cause severe dislocation not only in the family but throughout society. Society's response has not always been constructive. Fear, ignorance, and public bias have often combined to make absolutely miserable the experience of many families who confront the already overwhelming challenge of living with the presence of Huntington's disease. Rather than try to support and encourage these families, society has often contributed to their total disintegration. And this is not a thing of the past. It still goes on, even in the proudest and most advanced of countries. The time is at hand when social neglect can no longer be excused. Our inability, thus far, to defeat Huntington's disease itself is not matched by an inability to combat ignorance and cruelty. Not until those twin evils have been beaten can the many available means for improving the lot of Huntington's disease patients and their families be fully exploited.

9
Research Prospects

Research is the only hope they have to lift this black cloud hanging over their heads and give them hope.

The urgent and overwhelming plea from Huntington's disease patients and families across the nation is for increased support of biomedical research.

I think the essential point is that the time is right for Huntington's disease. More new possibilities for research have opened up in the last five years than in the previous one-hundred with respect to HD.

Everyone who is touched in any way by Huntington's disease is interested in medical research. Wherever HD families gather, people want to know about the state of contemporary research. What is known in the scientific community about this disease? How much attention is it receiving? Is money being appropriated to fund research? What is the most promising research? How close are we to a breakthrough? The hope sustaining many Huntingtonian families is that, one day, medical science will produce an explanation and a cure for the disease.

But some people put too much faith in scientific research. Young couples often discount the threat of Huntington's disease on the assumption that the disease will be cured by the time their children are old enough to begin showing symptoms. They proceed with a family as if the disease does not exist for them. Unfortunately, this is not a responsible attitude. We cannot lead our lives on the premise that solutions not available today are bound to exist in the near future. To do so can involve ourselves and our posterity in recurring tragedy. There were people in the 1940s and 1950s who had large families in the knowledge that their children might inherit the gene for Huntington's disease. Like many young people today, they rationalized that the disease would surely be conquered by the time their children reached maturity. Those children are now mature. Some of them have HD, and medical science is still a long way from being able to cure them.

Researchers working on a cure for Huntington's disease are confronted with a variety of problems. So little is understood about the fundamental cause of the disorder that it is difficult to know where to begin. If scientists knew more about the disease, they could focus their attention on the most promising leads. At our present state of knowledge, it is difficult to distinguish a false lead from one that might produce a breakthrough.

Scientists studying Huntington's disease are obliged to work in two areas that are at the far frontiers of human knowledge: the innermost workings of the human cell, and the way the brain functions. While it is true that more has been learned about Huntington's disease in the last five or ten years than in the whole previous history of the disorder, scientists are only now exploring the biomedical frontiers which may lead them to some definitive answers.

As noted in chapter 2, there is much about the human cell and the brain that remains a mystery. It is ironic that human beings can create great works of art, construct computers, and transport themselves to the moon while still understanding so little about the organ that makes it all possible. We do not know, for example, the precise brain mechanisms responsible for anger, joy, or other moods. We do not understand how memory works or exactly how thoughts are generated. Because Huntington's disease can affect mood, memory, and thought, some experts have concluded that HD research bears directly on "those areas of the brain that are least understood and quintessentially human."[1]

This is not to suggest that Huntington's disease is an impossible research problem or that it is being neglected. Until the 1960s, that statement could have been made with reasonable accuracy.

Much preliminary work had to be done in the general areas of genetics and neurology before scientists were in a position to begin asking some of the hard questions about Huntington's disease. But today HD and related disorders are receiving an enormous amount of attention. It would require many volumes to summarize the research projects currently underway. At a recent Huntington's disease symposium in San Diego, almost 100 scientific papers were presented.[2] Most of these papers reported on basic research on the cause, prevention, and treatment of HD. There are many other types of research as well. Elsewhere in this book, mention has been made of some of the research related to predictive testing, social adjustment, psychological reactions, and various forms of therapy. There are also research projects in progress concerning such various subjects as brain tissue banks, care centers, and supportive legislation.

Most of this research holds promise for improving the condition of those who are touched by HD. But the projects of greatest interest to the Huntingtonian family are those which seek to discover the underlying cause of the disease. Presumably, if scientists can understand what causes the disorder, they will be in a position to do something about it. This chapter focuses exclusively on a few of the main areas of inquiry which are aimed at unraveling the ultimate mysteries of Huntington's disease.

The material is presented in summary form only. It would be useless to the reader, and beyond the capacity of the author, to treat pertinent research in detail. Most of these areas are so complex that they require highly specialized training. The jargon in medical journals is by itself formidable enough to intimidate even the most dedicated lay reader. But the average person can understand the general areas of inquiry and some of the theories and assumptions upon which scientists are basing their investigations. That information is not only interesting, but encouraging, since it helps us to realize that significant scientific advances are being made. If there aren't many answers yet, at least much better questions are being asked. Perhaps the time *is* right for conquering Huntington's disease. Any one of the research directions sketched in this chapter may produce the breakthrough we all so fervently desire.

GENETICS

Chapter 2 focused on Huntington's disease as an autosomal dominant genetic disorder characterized by the loss of certain cells in the brain. The disease is inherited through our genes, which carry the biochemical code that dictates every human characteristic. Genetic research over the past decade indicates that a defective gene may produce a faulty protein, or protein product, which induces the cell degeneration responsible for the symptoms of Huntington's disease. Scientists are not absolutely certain that this hypothesis is correct, but there is considerable evidence in its favor. Where on the forty-six chromosomes of man the HD gene resides, however, is an unresolved question that must be investigated in further genetic studies.[3]

If all genetic conditions are, by their nature, very difficult to trace, the genetic transmission of HD does at least give researchers one advantage that they don't have in studying nongenetic neurological disorders. Research of nongenetic neurological diseases requires sampling of brain tissue, and since surgical biopsy performed on the brains of living subjects is often unacceptable, brain tissue for this research must usually be gotten from post-mortem sampling. Because HD is a genetic disorder, though, the mutant gene responsible for it can be presumed to abide in every cell of the body (since every cell possesses a full set of chromosomes and a full complement of genes). This being the case, it is possible to use easily obtainable skin cells (fibroblasts) or blood cells to investigate the origin of the disease.[4]

Once the genetic "trigger" is identified, researchers will be in a better position to understand how it fires the chemical bullets that kill certain cells. Identification of the gene locus will also help to explain why the HD gene usually does not take its toll until relatively late in life. If the defective gene is present from the moment of conception, why does it remain inactive until most carriers reach the fourth or fifth decade of life? Are there "modifier" genes nearby, holding the defective gene in check? Or is there perhaps some other force at work, such as a slow-acting virus? When the gene becomes active, precisely what biochemical changes occur? In seeking answers to these questions, scientists have achieved a fuller understanding of the biochemical basis of Huntington's disease.

BIOCHEMISTRY

Neurochemists are "chemists of the mind" who study the mechanisms of that marvelous universe called the human brain. Among their most exciting discoveries are a group of substances which act as chemical messengers within the brain. These are the neurotransmitters (mentioned at the conclusion of chapter 2), molecules that function between neurons to either initiate or inhibit specific actions. Neurochemists have begun to map the distribution of neurotransmitters in the brain, and to gain a better understanding of the brain's complex system of communication.[5]

It is widely believed that Huntington's disease may result from some disruption of the signals involved in this elaborate network of communication. Finding out exactly where and how this disruption occurs is not easy, but neurochemists have noted abnormalities in a number of neurotransmitter systems when HD is present. For example, the systems which utilize gamma-aminobutyric acid (GABA), acetylcholine, and substance P have all been implicated. Other neurotransmitter systems may also be involved; the total number of neurotransmitters in the human brain is not yet known.[6]

In this type of research the problem will probably not be so simple as identifying *the* neurotransmitter abnormality which is responsible for symptoms of Huntington's disease. The systems are too complex for that. A combination of systems which contribute to a delicate chemical balance may be involved. There are also other possibilities. For example, a neurotransmitter may be in short supply; or the enzyme that makes the neurotransmitter could be altered or missing; or the neurotransmitter receptors may be damaged so that neurons are unable to process chemical messages.

The pioneering research on GABA, an inhibitory neurotransmitter, conducted by Thomas L. Perry and others is discussed briefly in chapter 2. If it could be demonstrated that HD symptoms result from a deficiency of GABA, and a way could be found to raise GABA levels, then perhaps the effects of the disease could be mitigated or avoided. Working on this assumption, scientists like Perry have tried to find substances which would elevate GABA levels in the brain. So far they have met with only limited success, perhaps because the substances do not pass through the brain's blood barrier, or because the GABA receptors themselves are damaged in Huntington's disease.[7] Another possible reason why efforts to increase GABA neurotransmitter activity in the brain have failed to provide clinical improvement in patients with HD is that these treatments do not correct deficiencies of other neurotransmitters such as acetylcholine and substance P.

This brings us back to the question of whether decreased GABA levels and other neurotransmitter abnormalities are primary or secondary to the basic disease process. It now seems very likely that the apparent reduction of activity of GABA and other neurotransmitters simply reflects the death of neurons that use those neurotransmitters, while other neurons which use other neurotransmitters remain healthy. If so, how does the mutant gene for HD cause the death of certain populations of neurons? Are its effects confined to neurons, or does it affect cells elsewhere in the body?[8]

THE IMMUNE SYSTEM

The hypothesis that the prominent neurological symptoms in HD are effects of antecedent biological events occurring somewhere besides the brain itself cannot be discounted. One theory that draws on this hypothesis concerns the body's immune system. It is known that the body regularly produces antibodies to protect itself against infection and disease. This is the principle behind immunizations. By introducing a mild or low-level dosage of a toxin or pathogen, we encourage the body to produce specific antibodies which will safeguard it in case of serious exposures.

Occasionally, something goes wrong with the immune system. For example, the body may develop antibodies against itself. This is known as "autoimmunity." For reasons not completely understood, the body's immunological system fails to distinguish natural from invading substances and reacts against the former as if they were alien.[9] The result can be the destruction or partial destruction of some vital body process or organ. Experiments with mice, demonstrating that they live longer in a germ-free environment, suggest that the body's defense system may have something to do with the normal process of aging.[10] It may also be involved in the cause of Huntington's disease.

Norwegian and American scientists, working together, have discovered that patients afflicted with Huntington's disease often possess antibodies capable of damaging or destroying neurons. This does not necessarily mean that HD is an autoimmune disease, but it may mean that a specific immune response is generated against an agent found only in brains of HD patients. The nature of this agent and its relation to the HD gene remain to be determined.[11] Researchers in California have postulated that "there exists an HD immune response consisting of two components: a minor component directed against antigen common to all human brains, and a major component directed against antigen found thus far only in HD and MS [multiple sclerosis] brains."[12] The California scientists have also speculated that these responses may be linked to a viral involvement in HD. Viruses exist in which a DNA copy of the hereditary traits of the virus can integrate into the host chromosome and be inherited as a dominant gene, the products of which can be targets of the host immune system.[13] While this theory is far from proven, it remains an important area for research and affords opportunities to link research on Huntington's disease with work on other disorders, such as multiple sclerosis.

TRACE METALS

For many years, HD research proceeded on the reasonable assumption that this disorder must be roughly similar to other diseases which affected a certain portion of the brain known as the basal ganglia. When scientific advances were made in the understanding of Wilson's and Parkinson's diseases, it was naturally assumed that the first line of attack in HD research should be in the areas which had proven fruitful in work on the other disorders. Some points of similarity and difference between HD and Parkinson's disease have been cited; Wilson's disease is another useful case for comparison.

Wilson's disease is a late-onset, *recessive* disorder characterized by biochemical changes in the brain and degeneration of the liver. Many of its symptoms are strikingly similar to HD: awkward movements, garbled speech, diminished interest in personal appearance, unpredictable behavior, and so on. The disease was first described by Dr. S. A. Kinnier Wilson in 1912. As late as the 1940s, persons who inherited Wilson's disease eventually died from it because there was no effective treatment. After World War II, scientists discovered that the disease results from a genetically determined inability of the body to properly metabolize copper. Absence of the required gene leads to an excessive accumulation of copper in the liver and the brain. It also produces a greenish border that surrounds the cornea of each eye. This is called the "Kayser-Fleischer ring." It signals an excess of copper in the body, and is the most easily identified sign of the disease.[14]

The tide turned for patients with Wilson's disease in 1956 when Dr. John Walshe of Cambridge, England, discovered a new drug, penicillamine, which chelates copper, that is, forms a firm complex with copper and facilitates its eventual elimination from the body. Patients suffering from Wilson's disease were restored almost to normal when administration of penicillamine helped their bodies to handle copper properly. Achievements of this kind prompted scientists to investigate the possibility of trace metal abnormalities in other conditions.

Sometimes their work produced gratifying dividends. In 1972, for example, an English doctor, E. J. Moynahan, discovered that zinc taken orally restores the chemical balance necessary to remove most of the symptoms of a previously fatal disease known as "acrodermatitis enteropathica." Commenting on this achievement, Dr. Aubrey Milunsky has written, "A previously fatal genetic disease, while not cured, can be managed in such a way as to ensure a probable normal life expectancy, and this without even knowing the basic defect involved."[15]

This is the type of success that gives HD families real hope. If such breakthroughs can be achieved for other genetic disorders, then why not for Huntington's disease? There is no known reason why not, although it must be noted that most of the diseases which have yielded to treatment have been recessive rather than dominant disorders. It is also discouragingly true that the many experiments which have been conducted in an attempt to link HD with some abnormality in trace metals have all been unsuccessful.

In the 1950s some investigators believed that, like Wilson's disease, HD resulted from some dysfunction in the metabolism of copper. The theory was dropped when numerous experiments failed to prove its validity. Research then turned to other trace metals, such as manganese, iron, and lead, on the chance that one of them might be the culprit. In 1961, Professor Perry studied fourteen urinary trace metals in seven HD patients and nine normal control subjects. He came away with the conclusion that there was no significant difference. Later in the decade, Dr. Ntinos C. Myrianthopoulos and Dr. Benjamin Boshes conducted a similar study involving a large number of HD patients. They concluded, "The whole picture was one of hopeless inconsistency."[16]

Medical history is filled with breakthroughs that emerged in areas long considered hopelessly unproductive. The search for a trace metal abnormality in HD has not been abandoned. Special attention is still being given to the metabolism of calcium, manganese, copper, and zinc.[17] The release and uptake of neurotransmitters are linked to a correct balance of trace metals. It is not unreasonable to speculate that some defect in the body's metabolism of these metals, or perhaps an inability of cells to absorb them, is vitally significant in Huntington's disease.

CELL MEMBRANES

Trace metals may assume central importance in a disorder because of an inability of the cell to absorb and use them properly. Each cell is like a walled city. The outer wall is the cell membrane, which regulates what enters and leaves the cell. Certain molecules that span the cell membrane act as sentries, standing guard over the perimeter of the cell and monitoring each substance that seeks to enter or depart.[18] If something goes wrong with the sentries, substances which should be entering the cell might be excluded and others might be allowed to pass which would normally be kept out. The result could be cell death.

Some researchers believe that the key problem in Huntington's disease may be a defect in the cell membrane. Using advanced techniques such as electron spin resonance, scientists have noted subtle alterations in the physical and biochemical state of red blood cell membranes of patients with Huntington's disease.[19] Although preliminary reports conflict, other research suggests that similar membrane defects may be present in skin cells (fibroblasts) from HD patients.[20]

Professor Bruyn and others have also noted an apparent defect in the nuclear membrane of HD-affected neurons. There is a significant, slit-like indentation not found in any other disease. Another abnormality, Professor Bruyn has suggested, is a marked loss of the fibrous, nonnervous supporting elements (neuroglia) of the nervous system. He has postulated that the loss of these supporting fibers, which border all cavities of the brain and spinal cord, may reduce the body's ability to remove toxic compounds.[21]

ENDOCRINOLOGY

Some characteristics of Huntington's disease have incited suspicion that the body's endocrine system is at fault. The endocrine glands (for example the pancreas, pituitary, thyroid, parathyroid, adrenals, ovaries, and testes) secrete hormones into the bloodstream which interact with the central nervous system to regulate appetite, emotions, and various functions of the body. Some researchers are investigating the possibility that an abnormality in the secretion of certain hormones may set in motion a chain of biochemical events resulting in the symptoms of Huntington's disease.

Several avenues of research have opened up. One lead has been the discovery of abnormalities in the hypothalamus.[22] Another is the appearance in some HD patients of abnormal glucose tolerance and a resistance to insulin.[23] Researchers conducting independent investigations in a number of countries have also found alterations in the hormone that controls growth.[24] These findings, although still open to question (since some parallel research has yielded different results), tend to implicate the endocrine system. The still mysterious origins of many commonly observed characteristics of the disease might also conceivably involve the endocrine system. For example, the most obvious but as yet unproven explanation for the progressive weight loss experienced by most HD patients is the increased expenditure of calories due to involuntary muscle movement. But Dr. Edward D. Bird has noted weight loss in internal organs like the liver and kidneys.[25] Could it be that the cause of weight loss in HD patients is not just the obvious movement disorder, but a more subtle endocrine problem? Further study addressing this and other questions related to the interplay between the endocrine and nervous systems may shed significant light on the basic mechanisms of the disease.

DEFECTIVE DNA REPAIR

For lasting good health, we all require the ability to repair any damage that occurs to DNA, the genetic material in every cell nucleus which directs the production of countless essential enzymes and other proteins. Radiation, oxidizing agents, and many chemicals that we are constantly exposed to can damage DNA molecules. Normally, repair mechanisms correct minor injuries to DNA, or eliminate badly damaged DNA. However, in two serious hereditary disorders, xeroderma pigmentosum and ataxia telangiectasia, it is known that damage to DNA caused by exposure to ultraviolet light or ionizing radiation cannot be repaired properly. These two diseases are inherited in an autosomal recessive fashion, but the same type of error might occur in autosomal dominant disorders. Recently, scientists at the National Institutes of Health in the United States have shown that cultured lymphocytes (a kind of white blood cell) from HD patients are much more readily damaged by x-rays than are the lymphocytes of control subjects.[26] This raises the possibility that neurons in the brains of HD patients may die prematurely because the DNA in their nuclei is not properly repaired after damage by certain radiomimetic chemicals. Cells elsewhere in the body, such as blood cells and skin cells, are constantly reproducing, so that no one cell is required to function for very long, and a little damage to the DNA in a few cells may not matter very much. But neurons in the brain do not replace themselves. They must remain alive and healthy for at least seventy or eighty years. Damage to the DNA of many millions of neurons could be extremely harmful to normal brain function.

ANIMAL MODELS

An interesting feature of Huntington's disease is that it exists only in human beings. There is no comparable condition in animals. This places significant limits on the range of research. For many years, the disease could not be examined in animals, and drug trials had to be conducted with human beings because there was no animal model. If an animal model for the disease could be created, the scope of research would be greatly expanded. Animals, rather than humans, could be used to test new drugs and therapeutic ideas. Living tissue could be extracted from rats or mice more readily than from human patients. Furthermore, the ability to simulate the disease in animals should provide additional clues to its fundamental pathology.

In 1976, research teams developed what may prove to be a reliable animal model for the disease. The scientists sought a substance which, when injected into the brains of laboratory animals, would produce the types of neurotransmitter abnormalities that are believed to exist in Huntington's disease. They found it in a substance known as kainic acid.

By injecting kainic acid into certain areas of the brains of rats, the researchers were able to trigger changes which caused the animals to display symptoms similar to those seen in humans who have Huntington's disease. There were some significant differences. The behavioral and motor symptoms induced in the animals were not an exact replica of the disease in humans, and they were artificially produced rather than inherited. Nevertheless, the kainic acid model created interest as possibly the first biochemical model of certain features of Huntington's disease to be produced in other species.[27] Scientists now believe that it may be necessary to develop multiple animal models that will represent all stages of the disease. In an attempt to develop a better pharmacologic model, researchers in Illinois have altered the GABA content in the brain of laboratory rats. When this is done, the animals display certain characteristics, including choreic forepaw movements, similar to those observed in humans with Huntington's disease. Using these animals, the Illinois team is able to make trials of various drugs which may be useful in treating some symptoms of the disease.[28]

In addition to its obvious merits for therapeutic trials, the kainic acid animal model has produced other benefits. In its metabolic effects, kainic acid resembles glutamic acid, which appears to be a vital component in the human nervous system. An excess of glutamic acid can kill nerve cells in certain areas of the brain. In other words, in overabundance it can act as a neurotoxin. In 1976, P.L. and Edith McGeer reported from Vancouver that overactive glutamic acid-releasing neurons might underlie the cell degeneration in HD.[29] Scientists in other parts of the world are also trying to determine if raised glutamate levels may be a vital factor in bringing on the symptoms of Huntington's disease.[30]

CONCLUSION

This survey touches only briefly upon some of the main areas of inquiry in HD research, with the hope of giving the general reader a grasp of the essential problems and questions faced by researchers. The scientific task is obviously complex. There are no easy answers. It is quite understandable if people who are living from day to day with someone who is suffering from HD become impatient with the apparent inertia of scientific inquiry. Those who are unable to follow the medical literature, and that includes most of us, could easily conclude that nothing at all is being done. The slow and careful progress in the laboratory is not headline material.

While it is true that enough is never being done when it comes to conditions as serious as Huntington's disease, it is important for the concerned reader to know that many capable scientific teams are investigating this and related disorders. If governments were more generous with research appropriations, greater progress could be made. This would be a wise investment, because the current costs of the disease far exceed the amount provided for research.

Another problem which needs attention is the duplication of effort now characteristic of HD research. There is far too much overlapping research and insufficient coordination of information, both nationally and internationally. Time and precious resources are being wasted through the unnecessary duplication of experiments and trials. One possible model for a more logical and systematic approach to research is provided by the Quebec Cooperative Study of Friedreich's Ataxia.*

L'Association Canadienne de l'Ataxie de Friedreich was established almost single-handedly in 1973 by a courageous and determined man, Claude St-Jean. Despite the fact that he suffers from the disease, Claude St-Jean organized sixty Quebec clinicians and scientists, along with more than fifty patients, into a cooperative, multicenter, multidisciplinary attack on Friedreich's Ataxia. Dr. André Barbeau, of the Clinical Research Institute in Montreal, coordinated much of the scientific work, which began with a reassessment of all the known facts, opinions, and theories about the illness. The four medical schools in the Province of Quebec agreed to pool their resources and work under a common protocol. State-financed hospitalization and health insurance provided essential support, permitting the hospitalization and testing of volunteer patients without charge to them.

The scientific board that directed the project included in the protocol "every determination which has been claimed to be abnormal in Friedreich's Ataxia, even if based on a few cases and not confirmed."[31] The program got underway in October, 1974, when all sixty clinicians and scientists gathered for a three-day workshop to discuss and refine the protocol. Then the fifty

---

* Friedreich's Ataxia is a hereditary spinocerebellar degenerative disease beginning in childhood and characterized by degeneration of the lateral and posterior columns of the spinal cord, ataxia, speech disturbance, and a variety of other problems.

patients with Friedreich's Ataxia who had agreed to participate were divided into small groups and placed in hospital metabolic units, where each patient submitted to three or four weeks of extensive observation and tests. Testing began in October, 1974, and was finished in August, 1975. Screening tests were performed on every patient for each principal metabolic process implicated in Friedreich's Ataxia. A total of seventeen clinical, nine physiological, and thirty-two biochemical tests were included. A "standardization committee" was formed to compare and verify the methodologies employed in each research center. Then the arduous task of compiling the results began.

After the test results, records, reports, and statistics were organized, a series of weekend workshops was held to analyze and interpret the findings. The job of writing the material for publication was distributed among the participants. Initial findings were published in *The Canadian Journal of Neurological Sciences* in November, 1976. "Situation reports" of this type established "a base of verified physiological and biochemical facts from which to plan further investigations." The cooperative study then entered a sustained follow-up phase with additional reports published in the February, 1978, and May, 1979, issues of the same journal.

For a variety of reasons, Quebec offered an ideal location for a study of this type. But there is no reason why a similar effort could not be organized elsewhere for the study of Huntington's disease and related disorders. The "National Plan" suggested in the report of the U.S. Commission for the Control of Huntington's Disease represents a significant step in the right direction. Full implementation of this plan depends upon the awareness and support of members of Congress, federal and state authorities, the scientific community, and the interested public.[32] The challenge of formulating and implementing a coordinated *international* attack on Huntington's disease remains to be met.

At the conclusion of a chapter devoted to research on Huntington's disease, any author would be delighted to say with confidence that science is on the brink of the long-awaited breakthrough. To do that here would be misleading and dishonest. The research which has taken place, especially in the last decade, has yielded solid accomplishments and illuminated some vital questions. Prospects for the future are better now than at any other time in the history of the disease. But the road ahead will not be easy. Good counsel comes from Dr. I. S. Cooper, who has written, "False optimism can be just as dangerous as pessimism when judicious, commonsense approaches to a problem are what is needed."[33]

10
History

In the light of history the miseries of man become more human, more understandable. The failures of physicians and patients alike do not appear so useless, and when the overall picture is considered, signs of progress and improvement are more evident—a ray of hope is more justified.

With a powerful sweep of his father's arm, young George Huntington felt himself lifted from the ground to the hard, leather seat of the doctor's well-traveled, one-horse shay. The boy was excited. He enjoyed making the medical rounds with his father. As far back as he could remember, he had roamed the eastern end of Long Island when his father visited patients from East Hampton to Sag Harbor and from Amagansett to Bridgehampton.[1]

This particular day seemed ideal for a trip, but the elder Huntington drove the shay in moody and uncharacteristic silence. He was lost in thought about the state of the nation. He worried that the Democratic Party had fallen into total disarray in Charleston. Then the Republicans had nominated the rail-splitter from Sangamon County. The future appeared ominous. Who could say how the southern states would react if Lincoln won the election in November?

While the man worried about politics, the boy occupied himself with more useful things. He watched the horse work against its harness, and he studied the woods for a glimpse of a rabbit or a deer.

Father and son spent the morning making calls, farm to farm and village to village. Dr. Huntington would go into a house to visit his patient while young George sought ways to amuse himself. Soon the doctor's shrill whistle would alert both son and horse that it was time to move on to the next farm.

Toward midafternoon young George found the activity overtaking him. He grew drowsy in the warmth of the sun. His chin dipped to his chest and his body rolled gently to the rhythm of the horse's patient work. But then, suddenly, something happened which shook the boy wide awake and created an impression which he would not forget for the rest of his life.

Like apparitions from the forest, two women appeared on the road ahead. The women, whom George later learned were mother and daughter, approached the shay at a lurching gait which was so unsteady that the boy assumed they must be drunk. Both women were poorly dressed and pencil thin. They never stopped moving. It was as if all their muscles worked at once. Their heads bobbed and arms flailed the air as they weaved along the road. When they drew closer, George noticed that their faces formed grotesque and ever-changing expressions. To a young boy, they were an altogether startling sight.

As his father gently drew the horse to a stop, George recoiled in fright. His father placed a reassuring hand on the boy's knee and whispered that there was nothing to fear, then spoke to the women. They returned his greeting in garbled, unintelligible words. George was amazed that his father understood what they were trying to say. While the conversation continued, the boy concluded that the women must be possessed by an evil curse or demon. What else could make anyone act in this bizarre way?

After a brief talk, the doctor clucked to his horse and the shay moved slowly down the road. George turned to watch the women lurch along their way until they disappeared into the distance. Their image was printed indelibly on his mind.

A decade later, after he left home and moved west to establish a medical practice of his own in Ohio, twenty-two-year-old Dr. George Huntington remembered the incident as he prepared his historic paper, "On Chorea," for the Meigs and Mason Academy of Medicine in Middleport. Most of the paper, which was delivered on 15 February 1872, dealt with chorea minor, or Sydenham's chorea. Only in the final paragraphs did he describe in succinct and graphic language the chronic, hereditary chorea which had been explained to him by both his father and grandfather after their many years of experience with the disease on Long Island. Recalling his childhood experience, Huntington reported that the disease was viewed "with a kind of horror, and not at all alluded to except through dire necessity."[2]

The disease draws its contemporary name from Huntington because of his brief description of more than a century ago. Even though the disease bears his name, he was not the first to describe it. It might as justifiably have been called Elliotson's, Waters's, Wood's, Gorman's, Lyon's, or Lund's disease. Indeed, chronic, hereditary, adult chorea probably dates to ancient times. Certainly many people had reported it long before young Dr. Huntington presented his famous paper.

The word "chorea" is derived from Latin and Greek words pertaining to dancing, or a group of dancers. It was used in the medieval Latin expression *chorea sancti viti*, or St. Vitus's Dance, a term with specific reference to the epidemic dancing psychoses of the Middle Ages[3] which came to be applied to many conditions characterized by spasmodic muscular contractions. The exact origin of the term is unclear. One stage of its derivation is evident: in 1418, at Strasbourg, St. Vitus (an early Christian martyr) was named protector of persons troubled by the dancing plague. But the remoter derivation of the term may be from June dances honoring the Slavonic sun-god Swantewit, for whose name the church may have substituted St. Vitus's in order to switch the emphasis from a pagan to a Christian theme.[4]

Many factors are thought to have contributed to the dancing mania—among them, persecution, natural and man-made disasters, and religious hysteria. In some instances, Sydenham's chorea may have been involved. It is more benign than Huntington's chorea and is neither chronic nor progressive. The quick, involuntary muscle movements in Sydenham's chorea often follow a streptococcal infection, and usually disappear completely with time.[5]

Whatever the malady, for centuries people with involuntary muscle movements or frantic behavior were thought to be possessed by evil spirits or demons. It is believed, for example, that at least one of the alleged "witches" executed in Salem, Massachusetts, in the 1690s suffered from Huntington's chorea.[6] One nineteenth-century authority reported that some people he knew explained the disease as a visitation upon those whose ancestors had reviled and mimicked Jesus of Nazareth while he was on the cross.[7] This is a particularly alarming and cruel example of the stigmatization that people with the disorder have had to endure for centuries. Readers who have had a long association with Huntington's disease and the public prejudices so often associated with it may sometimes feel that society has not come all that far since these abusive notions were prevalent. Sufferers of neurological disease are no longer executed for witchcraft, but a significant segment of the public still acts as if the mentally handicapped are cursed or possessed by devils.

Use of the word *chorea* to describe a specific, organic disorder has been attributed to Paracelsus (1493–1541) in the sixteenth century. He struggled to differentiate various types of the disease and check the indiscriminate use of the term St. Vitus's Dance.[8] Other writers made note of various forms of chorea throughout the seventeenth and eighteenth centuries, but the scientific classification of what is now called Huntington's disease dates from the nineteenth century.[9]

References to "adult chorea" abound in early nineteenth century British medical literature, but perhaps the first published description was Dr. John Elliotson's essay, "St. Vitus' Dance," in the inaugural issue (1832) of the British medical journal, *Lancet*.[10] This account appeared forty years before Huntington's celebrated paper. In 1841 Dr. C. O. Waters of Franklin, New York, reported on what is now known as Huntington's disease, describing details of cases which Huntington himself may have seen in the same area years later. In Waters's time, the disease was locally referred to as "the magrums."[11]

In 1846, Dr. Charles R. Gorman reported from Pennsylvania that hereditary chorea was more prevalent in that state than anyone had supposed. A few years later, Dr. George B. Wood of the University of Pennsylvania described a case of "aggravated chorea, which resisted *all* treatment."[12] Nor was the disease recognized only in adults. In 1863, Dr. Irving W. Lyon of Bellevue Hospital in New York reported three patients with hereditary chorea, one of whom was the first juvenile case on record.[13]

Studies of the disease were also made in countries other than the United States and England. Throughout the 1850s and 1860s, a district physician, Dr. J. C. Lund, reported on cases of hereditary chorea in Norway. Professor George W. Bruyn has suggested that hereditary chorea might now be properly known as Lund's disease if Norwegian had been as popular as English. In Scandinavia the disease is, in fact, sometimes referred to as Lund-Huntington's chorea.[14]

Other credits notwithstanding, it was Huntington's concise description of the disease that determined its contemporary name. There have never been any serious moves to change it. In recent years the term *Huntington's chorea* has been modified to simply *Huntington's disease* because not all persons with the disease display choreic symptoms. One authority on the early history of the disease paid tribute to those who contributed descriptions before Dr. Huntington's, but then concluded, "It would be churlish to quibble about the name of the disease which, if historically inaccurate, has the advantage of being universally recognized."[15]

Summaries of the recent history of Huntington's disease raise some interesting questions. If the disease did not suddenly appear from nowhere in the nineteenth century, what can be learned of its activity before the descriptions published between 1832 and 1872? The ancient references are limited and not specific. Why is there so little mention of the disease before the nineteenth century? Hasn't the disorder passed from one generation to the next for many centuries?

It must be remembered that systematic, scientific methodology was only in its infancy in the eighteenth and nineteenth centuries. Many who practiced medicine were poorly trained and even illiterate. Carefully recorded observations were the exception rather than the rule. More important, perhaps, the nature of heredity was not clarified until Mendel's famous plant experiments in the 1860s. And Mendel's pioneering achievements did not become widely known until after they were rediscovered around 1900.[16] Before that, Huntington's disease was present but misdiagnosed, poorly understood, and usually unrecorded.

There is a less obvious reason why the disease was not clearly apparent before the middle of the nineteenth century. In a manner of speaking, it was present but invisible. Hereditary adult chorea existed in those days, but the shorter life expectancy meant that many people who carried the gene did not live long enough for symptoms to become apparent. As carriers of the gene, they passed the risk to their children, but often died from other causes before they were themselves old enough to suffer any effects. As one authority put it, "Prevailing conditions in the past concealed the florid picture of the inherited disease."[17]

The situation began to change as modern science enabled human beings to enjoy a longer average life span. With people living longer, Huntington's disease had more time to take its toll. This was illustrated in a comparative study undertaken by Dr. David L. Stevens of Leeds Hospital in England. He examined the frequency of Huntington's disease in the general population of England and Wales in 1966 and compared those statistics to figures for 1841, the earliest year in which reliable demographic information was available. The general population was much younger in 1841, because the average life expectancy at birth was only 40.2 years for males and 42.2 years for females. By 1966 the figures were 68.4 years and 74.7 years respectively. By applying statistical analysis to the life expectancy figures and the incidence of observed chorea, Stevens deduced that the frequency of those who *carried* the gene for HD was about the same in 1841 as it was in 1966, but the frequency of those who actually *expressed* symptoms was much less. He concluded:

> In 1841 there were far more unaffected carriers of the gene than choreics, a fact clearly illustrated by the ratios of unaffected carriers to choreics—2.85 in 1841 and 1.62 in 1966. These differences, which are entirely due to the different expectation of life, and, therefore, the different age structure of the population, offer a ready explanation for the apparent rarity of the disease, and a possible explanation for the failure of recognition of its hereditary nature in the early part of the nineteenth century. The gene that causes the disease was no less common than it is now, but fewer carriers of this gene lived long enough to develop chorea. Consequently, even those who survived long enough to reproduce may often have died before they had themselves manifested the disease that they had transmitted to their offspring, which would tend to conceal the hereditary nature of the condition and would cause the fairly frequent appearance of individuals with chronic incurable chorea, but no apparent family history of the condition.[18]

European carriers of the defective gene spread the disease around the globe when the Americas, Australia, and other areas were colonized. In 1932, Dr. P. R. Vessie tracked the majority of cases in New England to three persons who emigrated to America in 1630 from the tiny village of Bures in East Anglia. Vessie traced almost one thousand cases spanning twelve generations and three centuries.[19] His work is still frequently cited as the authoritative reference on the introduction of Huntington's disease into America.

In 1969, researchers at the Veterans Administration Hospital in Albany, New York, challenged the accuracy of Vessie's paper. While tracing the family history of a seventy-seven-year-old patient admitted to their care in 1966, Mary Hans and Dr. Thomas H. Gilmore concluded that there were significant inaccuracies in Vessie's work. Researchers in England and else-where reached the same conclusion. Narrowing the field of inquiry to the Bures group, Hans and Gilmore suggested, is not justified. They noted the existence of several Huntingtonian families dating to colonial times, described as being "distin-guished by a tendency to inter-marriage and a generousness in perpetuating Huntington's chorea."[20]

The origin of the disease in other countries has received close scrutiny. Professor André Barbeau led one team which traced 173 cases in Quebec to a woman who emigrated from France to Montreal in 1645.[21] In 1934 McDonald Critchley performed a similar service, outlining the natural history of Huntington's disease in East Anglia.[22] Dr. C. R. D. Brothers, director of mental hygiene in Tasmania, published a brief but fascinating article in 1949 concerning the origin of the disorder in that part of Aus-tralia.[23]

Studies by Brothers, A. W. Meadows, Betty Teltscher, and others revealed that a woman, believed to be of French descent, arrived in Tasmania aboard the *Arab* in 1842. She came with her second husband and her eight children. After settling in northeast Tasmania, she had five more children. This woman carried the gene for Huntington's disease. From among her thirteen children, five of the six females and four of the seven males inherited the disorder. Her descendants crossed Bass Strait and carried the gene to other parts of Australia.[24]

It is possible, of course, that Huntington's disease existed in

Australia and the Americas among the aboriginal populations before the arrival of Europeans. Australian Aborigines, justifiably suspicious after two centuries of exploitation by Europeans, are reluctant to volunteer sensitive personal information of this type for fear that it will be used against them. One careful study of Huntington's disease in a South Australia community of Aboriginal descent indicated that the disorder was introduced into the Aboriginal population in 1867 by a European male who carried the defective gene.[25]

In some countries, state-by-state or province-by-province surveys have been conducted in an effort to identify every case of the disease. In 1969–70, for example, the late Dr. David C. Wallace completed for the Australian state of Queensland a study begun by Dr. Neville Parker many years before. An attempt was made "to ascertain and to study every diagnosed case of the disease in Queensland, and to obtain details concerning the family history in every instance."[26] Similar work has been completed in Victoria and in states and provinces of other countries.

When his data were tabulated, Dr. Wallace found that the incidence of the disease in Queensland was higher than had been thought. This seems to be a general rule wherever statistics on HD are carefully collected. For example, after reviewing published surveys in the early 1970s, researchers at Creedmoor State Hospital in Queens Village, New York, concluded that the prevalence of the disease is "quite probably higher than has been previously estimated, at least in the New York area."[27]

Because the disease has been so heavily stigmatized, a conspiracy of silence masks its true incidence and makes it appear rarer than it actually is. In Queensland, Dr. Wallace estimated "a frequency of one overt case of Huntington's chorea per 15,800 persons, or 6.3 per 100,000, and a frequency of carriers of the abnormal gene of one per 5,700 of the population or 17.7 per 100,000."[28] He concluded that "perhaps 7 to 7.5 per 100,000 represents the true incidence in most large populations of European descent."[29]

In certain relatively isolated geographical locations, "circumstances have contributed to endemic levels of astonishing magnitude, such as 51.9 per 100,000 near Maracaibo in Venezuela and 560 per 100,000 for the Moray Firth area in Scotland."[30] The disease was probably introduced into the Venezuelan state of

Zulia on the western shores of Lake Maracaibo in the 1860s by a sailor aboard a German trade ship. Many of the descendants of a liaison between the sailor and a local inhabitant developed the disease.[31]

In 1973, Dr. K. W. G. Heathfield published the following prevalence reports from around the world:

Table of Prevalence

Country	Area	Authors	Year	Prevalence 100,000
Australia	Tasmania	Brothers	1949	17.4
	Victoria	Brothers	1964	4.8
	Queensland	Parker	1958	2.3
		Wallace & Parker	1972	6.3
Canada	Quebec	Barbeau (Myrianth-opoulos, 1966)	1964	2.4
Germany	Rhineland	Panse	1938	3.2
Japan	Aichi	Kishimoto	1959	0.4
Spain	Cadiz	Ordonez	1970	1.4
U.K.	London	Minski & Guttman	1938	1.8
England	Northampton	Oliver	1970	6.3
		Pleydell	1955	6.5
	Bedfordshire	Heathfield & McKenzie	1971	7.5
	Essex (NEMRHB)	Heathfield	1967	2.5
	Leeds	Stevens	1972	4.3
	Cornwall	Bickford & Ellison	1953	5.6
Scotland	Southwest	Bolt	1970	5.6
	Moray Firth	Lyon	1962	560.0
U.S.A.	Minnesota	Person et al.	1955	5.4
	Michigan	Reed & Chandler	1958	4.1
	Rochester (Minn.)	Kurland	1968	6.7
Venezuela		Negrete (Went, 1972)	1970	"very high"

Source: K. W. G. Heathfield, "Huntington's Chorea: a centenary review," *Postgraduate Medical Journal* 49 (Jan. 1973), p. 41.

VOLUNTARY HEALTH ORGANIZATIONS

The United States

Perhaps the most exciting and productive development in the recent history of the struggle against Huntington's disease has been the growth of private health organizations devoted to promoting research, improving conditions for patients, and raising public awareness about neurological illness. These organizations rely primarily on the services of volunteers, including people with neurological illness, those who may be at risk for genetic disorders, relatives concerned about these diseases, medical professionals, and persons who are simply interested in devoting their time and skills to a worthwhile effort. Readers who are not already involved and who have some time to invest wisely may wish to contact their nearest HD group for more information. Addresses and phone numbers of organizational headquarters are listed in appendix 2.

The work of the private health organizations has done much to revolutionize both scientific and public attitudes toward Huntington's disease. The new era began in 1967, the year in which a remarkable woman saw her legendary husband die from the effects of the disorder. Marjorie Guthrie later wrote about her final visit with Woody:

> On his dying day he heard us come into his room, opened his eyes, and made a grunting sound when I asked him if he would like some water. I fed him a spoon of water to wet his dry lips. He was still a whole person, but this person was dying and he knew it. We knew it too, and the hospital chaplain who was standing by asked if he might say a prayer. He recited the Lord's Prayer, and we all looked at each other, listening quietly. I told the chaplain that Woody had always loved to read the Bible and was more versed in the Bible than most people. He had always enjoyed studying the religions of the world, and throughout this conversation he was listening with his eyes sometimes closed and sometimes open. When I left the hospital, I stroked his forehead. I knew it was the last time.[32]

Long before Woody died, Marjorie had begun to ask what could be done about Huntington's disease. She turned to Dr. John Whittier with the plea, "Please, educate me. I want to do something about this devastating hereditary illness." She found three other families affected by Huntington's disease, and began to reach out looking for more. From that small beginning grew the Committee to Combat Huntington's Disease (CCHD). CCHD now has forty chapters in the United States, a mailing list of more than 20,000 names, and a worldwide outreach.

After Woody Guthrie's death, his friends gathered in Carnegie Hall for a benefit concert. The money collected from this and other fund-raising ventures enabled Marjorie to attack a variety of objectives: developing CCHD; providing support to neurologists, biochemists, and other researchers; recruiting skilled minds for the struggle against the disease; reducing the stigma attached to the disease; encouraging patients and those at risk to join the fight; informing politicians and public health authorities; and harnessing the enormous energies of the interested public who had no way to participate in the collective effort to conquer HD and related disorders.

Marjorie soon met Dr. Ntinos Myrianthopoulos of the National Institutes of Health (NIH) in Bethesda, Maryland, near Washington, D.C. As a leader in the scientific struggle against the disease, Dr. Myrianthopoulos had published a review article in 1966 summarizing the "state of the art" with regard to Huntington's disease. He was also helping to organize the first workshop on HD at the 1967 meeting of the World Federation of Neurology. Marjorie's determination to promote new interest in the disorder coincided with scientific initiatives which promised fresh hope for progress. The old regime of fear and hopelessness was about to give way to a new age of bold activity.

With the support of Creedmore Hospital in New York, and on the recommendation of Secretary of the Interior Stewart Udall, Marjorie was able to assure additional NIH support for Dr. Myrianthopoulos and the Huntington's disease workshop. She then went to the World Federation of Neurology conference in Montreal and asked the scientists gathered there what more she could do. They replied that they needed someone who could help bring Huntington's disease out of hiding. Families had concealed the disorder for centuries. HD research would not be successful as long as individuals and families were either afraid or had no opportunity to come forward and participate in the struggle against the disorder. The treatment of patients could not be improved, and public awareness would not be increased, as long as Huntington's disease and other neurological illnesses were hidden from view. Much needed to be done to remove the stigma from HD and counter the bias against the neurologically handicapped which existed in public attitudes and the law.

The scientists had turned to the right person. A professional dancer, and former first assistant in the Martha Graham School of Dance, Marjorie Guthrie brought boundless energy to the task. Every year she logs tens of thousands of miles organizing and promoting the crusade against Huntington's disease and other genetic and neurological disorders. She appears on radio and television, before various legislative bodies, and in scientific meetings. She is a consultant for more than a dozen different health groups. In 1977 she chaired the U.S. Commission for the Control of Huntington's Disease and Its Consequences, which was established by the 94th Congress under Public Law 94-63.

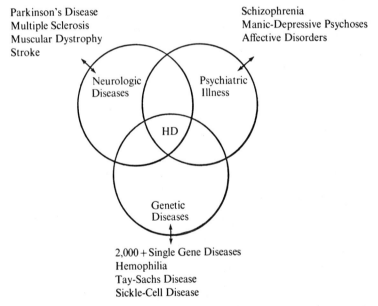

Figure 10.1. Huntington's disease as a prototype for research and treatment of other neurologic, psychiatric, and genetic diseases. From *Report: Commission for the Control of Huntington's Disease and Its Consequences*, vol. 1 (Bethesda, Md.: National Institutes of Health, 1977).

Under Marjorie's leadership, along with that of Executive Director Dr. Nancy S. Wexler and others, the Commission "made national health history . . . by recommending a concerted attack by the Federal government on the basic biomedical research that relates to any neurologic, psychiatric, and genetic disorder, as well as chronic disease, *not just* Huntington's disease."[33] The three interlocking circles depicted on the preceding page represent the Commission's goal of serving "the interests and needs of more than one group of patients . . . so that the plan can benefit millions of Americans."[34] As this book went to press, Marjorie Guthrie was instrumental in persuading Congress to increase funding by $30 million to the National Institute of Neurological and Communicative Disorders and Stroke. Some of this money will be used to implement the national plan recommended by the Commission.

In addition to making a broad range of recommendations for government involvement, the Commission served to coordinate the efforts of all the voluntary Huntington's disease organizations in America, including the Hereditary Disease Foundation, the National Huntington's Disease Association, and the Huntington's Chorea Foundation.

The Hereditary Disease Foundation was founded in California in 1974. It had its roots in the California Committee to Combat Huntington's Disease, but reorganized as a separate foundation to facilitate its support for basic scientific research in genetics. Under the leadership of Dr. Milton Wexler and a board of trustees and scientific advisors with a wide range of expertise, the Hereditary Disease Foundation pours 90 percent of all its proceeds into direct support for genetic research. HDF also sponsors interdisciplinary workshops aimed at generating new ideas for investigation, and publishes a series of "Workshop Notebooks" which are distributed to more than 250 researchers throughout the world.[35]

Like HDF, the National Huntington's Disease Association (NHDA) had its roots in the Committee to Combat Huntington's Disease. NHDA was founded in April, 1976, by three chapters which had been part of CCHD. By 1979 it had developed eleven chapters of its own, along with twenty area representatives throughout the country. Heavily committed to research support,

NHDA allocated more than $50,000 for that purpose between 1976 and 1979. It has budgeted another $39,000 to fund research in 1980.[36]

The Huntington's Chorea Foundation (HCF) was chartered in Houston, Texas, in 1967. Mrs. Alice Pratt, who subsequently served on the executive board of the Commission for the Control of Huntington's Disease, was primarily responsible for establishing HCF. By the end of 1979, HCF had poured $1,000,000 into basic research on Huntington's disease. HCF research grants in 1979 totaled $107,000, and chiefly supported work investigating the role of neurotransmitters in HD. Among many other projects, HCF contributed to the funds which led to Dr. Edward D. Bird's establishment of brain tissue banks in England and America. In 1979 HCF was dissolved, and its funding efforts were assumed by the Wills Foundation, with headquarters in Houston.[37]*

England

The establishment of the Committee to Combat Huntington's Disease in the United States inspired the formation of similar groups in other countries. Both England and Canada owe the development of their HD organizations to the work of Marjorie Guthrie and the determination of private citizens in those countries.

The Association to Combat Huntington's Chorea (COMBAT) was established in 1971 after its current national secretary, Mrs. Mauveen Jones, contacted Marjorie Guthrie for information and assistance. A few years earlier, a medical specialist in London had informed Mrs. Jones that only about a dozen British families were affected by Huntington's disease. It is now known that there are approximately 6,000 HD patients in Britain.

Through the good offices of a newspaper, Mrs. Jones invited HD families to contact her. Seventy-six families responded to that invitation. From this beginning, COMBAT has grown to twenty-three branches, twelve area representatives, and a full-time staff of four. The organization is funded by a grant from the

* The Wills Foundation, P.O. Box 66704, Houston, Texas 77006; phone (713) 965-9043.

Department of Health and Social Security (a projected £15,000 in 1980), a £5,000 annual gift from Marks & Spencer Ltd. stores, and donations contributed twice yearly from the various COM-BAT branches. COMBAT produces an informative newsletter, conducts an extensive public education program, and sponsors a holiday home, a family counseling service, and a broad range of scientific research. During 1977–79 COMBAT supported more than a dozen research projects with grants totaling about £40,000.[38]

Canada

The Huntington Society of Canada began when a school counselor, Ralph Walker, discovered that some of the youngsters in his school were at risk for the disease. With relatives of his own at risk, Ralph concluded that HD was not rare at all, but hidden by most families. Ralph and his wife, Ariel, decided to devote their spare time to organizing some of these families. A request to Marjorie Guthrie brought them prompt and enthusiastic assurance of support from CCHD in the United States. The McMaster Medical School in Hamilton also offered assistance. In October, 1973, Marjorie flew from New York to Toronto to be present at the first public meeting of the new Huntington's disease society. The Walkers had hoped that thirty or forty people might attend. Instead, 150 were present. Letters began to arrive from all across Canada from people who were concerned about the disease.

By the end of 1975, the Huntington Society of Canada had received its Letters Patent and was registered as a Canadian charitable organization. In 1977 the Society moved from the Walkers' home into an office building in Cambridge, Ontario. In 1980 it had a national staff of four and more than twenty chapters and branches in seven of the ten Canadian provinces. The Society offered its first predoctoral research scholarships in 1977, its first postdoctoral fellowship in 1979, and its first operating grants in 1980. In addition to support for research, it is committed to educational programs for HD families, the medical and scientific communities, and the general public. The Society has also initiated a brain tissue donation program and works to find and develop services required by individuals suffering from the disease.[39]

Australia

For many years the most original and vigorous research on Huntington's disease in Australia has come from the University of Melbourne's Department of Psychiatry. Dr. Colin Brackenridge led a team of enterprising workers in wide-ranging epidemiological and statistical investigations. By 1972, Brackenridge, Professor Brian Davies, Dr. Edmond Chiu, and Betty Teltscher, a research social worker, had begun preparation for the establishment of the Australian Huntington's Disease Association.

When both the research and organizational aspects of the work had reached their most promising stage, the Australian government, which has never been generous in its allocations for medical research, withdrew the supporting grant. A private benefactor came forward with a substantial contribution to keep the work going for another year, but it was soon clear that the Australian effort would die in its infancy unless substantial support could be found. The government seemed content to ignore the plight of approximately 1,200 Australians who suffered from the disease and the many thousands more who were either at risk or otherwise influenced by the disorder.

A public meeting was called at the University of Melbourne to discuss the crisis. Derek Scales, a Melbourne advertising and publicity agent, moved that plans proceed with the formation of an Australian Huntington's Disease Association (AHDA). If the government would not support the effort, then the AHDA would raise funds, support research, help individuals and families, educate the medical profession, and do whatever it could to support hospitals and other institutions charged with the care of HD patients.

Soon news of the Association began to spread, and letters arrived from all over Australia, written by concerned citizens who thought that they alone faced the many problems associated with Huntington's disease. Within a few years AHDA chapters were formed by private citizens in every one of Australia's six states. In November, 1979, representatives from each of those chapters, along with delegates from the Australian Capital Territory, New Zealand, Canada, the Netherlands, and the United States gathered in Melbourne for the first AHDA national conference. The conference venue was the magnificent five-acre estate known as Mary's Mount which forms the real-life setting for the fictionalized experiences of Ian Miller in the first chapter of this book.

The Australian Huntington's Disease Care Centre at Mary's Mount is the first facility of its type in the world. It promises to serve as a model for the management of the disease. It primarily serves HD patients who are residents of the state of Victoria, but there is a constant liaison between the AHDA in Victoria and chapters in other states. There is also a separate, seaside "holiday home" for HD patients in Victoria, and persons suffering from the disease have travelled from other states to enjoy this vacation opportunity.[40]

Belgium

In 1974 the "Huntington League" was created in Flanders, the Dutch-speaking northern half of Belgium. The League is composed of dozens of families, working together on a voluntary basis to bring information, professional support, ethical discussions, and research encouragement to the struggle against the disease. The League aims at *primary* prevention, by encouraging individuals to act voluntarily to prevent the disease from being passed to future generations; *secondary* prevention, by detecting and treating the disorder as early as possible; and *tertiary* prevention, by preventing the patient and family from suffering unnecessary handicaps related to HD such as a premature loss of work, social stigma, and severe depression. Leuven, Belgium, was the setting for an international congress of HD family organizations in September, 1981.[41]

International Huntington's Disease Association

The work of voluntary health associations devoted to the struggle against HD is not limited to the countries discussed above. The effort is genuinely international. Unfortunately, space does not permit a detailed examination of the HD association in every country. In addition to the groups already mentioned, associations have been formed in France, Italy, Spain, New Zealand, and a number of other countries.

In August, 1974, representatives from HD organizations in the

United States, Canada, Australia, Belgium, and Britain formed the International Huntington's Disease Association as a means of bringing together the rapidly growing national groups.[42] Fortunately, this type of international exchange is commonplace in the scientific community. The rapid growth of interest in HD research is illustrated by the two major international symposiums on the disease held during the past decade. The 1972 Centennial Symposium on Huntington's Disease took place in Columbus, Ohio, and the Second International Symposium convened in San Diego, California, in 1978. A forging together of scientific activity and lay interest can make a formidable weapon against HD. It is through this collective effort that the day will come when Huntington's disease enters the pages of history as an illness which no longer threatens mankind.

Reference Matter

Appendix 1

Caring for the HD Patient at Home

The following practical hints on caring for the HD patient at home were prepared by the Department of Health, State of New York, in conjunction with the Committee to Combat Huntington's Disease.

Living with HD will undoubtedly be stressful to all members of the family. As long as the HD patient remains at home, there is good evidence that the suggestions given below may strengthen the family relationships and contribute to the well-being of each member.

EXERCISES

Encourage daily exercising and walking as long as possible. Allow time for frequent rests. Exercising on a mat with recorded music makes movement pleasurable. Organize a set routine for each day. Exercise is an important factor in maintaining good general health.

Head: When the patient is lying face up, use a pillow to protect the head; when sitting, prop head or incline chair to support in comfortable position. Have patient practice lifting head up and down while lying on stomach; while sitting, patient can practice lifting and rotation.

Eyes: Place your hand 12″ in front of and in line with patient. Ask patient to follow movement of your hand with his/her eyes. Move hand toward right shoulder, stop, back to midline, stop, then to left shoulder, stop, back to midline, stop—repeat.

Breathing: Encourage patient to inhale deeply and blow air out slowly while lying on back. Repeat sitting upright.

Arms, Shoulders, Hands, Fingers: While holding his/her hands, help patient pull up and down. Suggest tighter hand grips. Have patient extend and cross arms, circle shoulders and wrists, open and close fingers.

Legs, Knees, Feet: Movements patient can practice: While lying on back, spread legs, then bring them together. With legs slightly spread, turn knees in and out. Lift and lower legs singly and together. Bend knee to chest and lower. Rotate ankles. Flex heels, pulling toes up and down.

Walking: Have patient practice walking forward, backward, side step; alone or with assistance if needed.

Transferring off Chair: Teach patient to assist moving from bed to chair by using pull rope or hand rail. Correct bed height; position chair to side of patient's strength. With or without help, patient should be out of bed daily.

DAILY TASKS

Dressing: Use elasticized waistbands on underwear and pants. Sew velcro tape (purchased in fabric shops) to replace buttons. Boots are easy to slip on and off. Use loose, unrestrictive clothing that is washable and doesn't need ironing.

Bathroom: Provide armchair or wall rails where possible. Foam rubber over HOT and COLD tap levers makes turning water off and on easier. Allow patient privacy for toilet needs. Use protective pants for incontinence.

Homemaker Aid: Large pockets in aprons can carry needed items.

Cosmetics: Tape foam rubber on small cosmetic tubes and containers for easier grasping and manipulation.

Sleeping: Pad footboards, headboards and railings around hospital or conventional beds. When necessary, a mattress on the floor surrounded by pillows can be a safe, comfortable bed. Use sleeping bag zipped around patient for blanket.

Shaving: Use electric or battery razor.

Protection: Padding made from fake sheepskin can be wrapped around rubbed, raw skin. Sheepskin mitts and stockings can cover extremities. Lightweight foam helmets can protect heads.

Smoking: Use "robot" smoker which patient smokes through a long tube while cigarette is held safely on table. Try to eliminate smoking.

TREATMENT

Experimental Medication: There is no one proven special treatment for HD at this time. There are, however, a number of experimental medications that help control some of the involuntary movements of some patients, and others that alleviate the depression and irritability which affect many HD patients.

Adjusting Medication: The family physician and neurologist may prescribe several drugs to be given in varying amounts, at various times, according to the special needs of each patient. Over and under medication may occur, requiring adjustments of dosages.

Side Effects: Sometimes a patient does not respond well to the prescribed medication, perhaps experiences increased movement, greater depression, restlessness, inability to sleep. When undesirable side effects are reported, the physician may change the medication.

Response of Symptoms: A "good" response means more control of involuntary movements, better emotional control, improved speech, and the ability of the patient to function better on a day-to-day basis. Even though HD cannot be cured, its progress can be slowed down.

COMMUNICATION

Patients become irritable and depressed when verbal communication becomes difficult. PATIENCE and good listening habits are the keys to assist the patient and avoid increased anxiety and agitation.

Patient and family should plan methods of communication, other than verbal communication, *before* difficult situations occur.

Speech: Speech is affected because of inability to control respiration, phonation, and articulation. Sounds like "L" and "N" are difficult and require special exercises. Speech and music therapy to educate the patient and family are highly recommended.

Encourage talking! Help patients by listening. Ask them to repeat carefully words that are not understandable.

There are other methods: Use a picture chart for patient to identify common needs, such as cold, hunger, blanket, bathroom, TV, yes, no, etc.

Many patients remain alert long after speech becomes difficult. Include patient in family discussions and social activities. Even with a limited response capability the patient wants to, and can, contribute to conversations. No one wants to be forgotten or ignored!

NUTRITION

Planned Diet: Good nutrition is essential to maintain the HD patient, especially to counteract the aging process.

Supplemental Vitamins: Daily:
   Vitamin E (400 units)
   Vitamin C (500 units)
   Vitamin B-1 complex (1 tablet)

What to Avoid:
   Deep fried foods
   Alcoholic beverages
   [Foods which are difficult to swallow]
Eating Tips: Because swallowing is difficult and choking is a common problem, keep a watchful eye during meals.
   Use adjustable height table over bed or chair.
   Tape foam rubber around handles of utensils for easier holding.
   Strap spoon to wrist.
   Use flexible straws, two-handled plastic mug, or cut a hole in the tight-fitting lid of a Tupperware spill-proof plastic glass for easier drinking.
   Prepare soft foods, milkshakes, blended mixtures; cut small portions of solids; crush crackers and breads into liquids.
   Suction cups can keep items from slipping. Rubber soap dish holders with suction cups will steady dishes.

WORK, RECREATION, RESPITE CARE

Work Ability: Many patients CAN and should be encouraged to do useful work such as gardening, simple household chores (collecting laundry from washing machine, painting large areas that do not require finite movement, collecting wood for fire, and washing unbreakable dishes). Being responsible at the appropriate level helps the patient maintain a positive self-image.

Hobbies: Listening to favorite records, singing, developing hobbies, making gifts from wood, tile and leather, or arts and crafts can be fun for many.

Recreation: Include the patient when the family plans picnics, rides, visits to local sports events or motion pictures. Interaction with other members of the family and neighborhood is important.

Respite Care: Every member of the HD family needs a break from the strain of caring for an HD patient. A program of placing a home-bound patient in a complete care facility for a week or so is being developed . . . (contact your local HD organization).

EMERGENCIES

SOS Card: Prepare a large SOS sign to be displayed in a prominent place, slipped under a door, or placed where another person would see that help is needed.

Medic Alert: Provide a MEDIC ALERT or similar identification to be worn by the patient.

Appendix 2

Addresses of Huntington's Disease Organizations

Committee to Combat Huntington's Disease
250 W. 57th St., Suite 201, New York, New York 10019.
Phone: (212) 757-0443.

The Hereditary Disease Foundation
9701 Wilshire Blvd., Suite 1204, Beverly Hills, California 90212.
Phone: (213) 274-5443.

National Huntington's Disease Association
Suite 501, 1441 Broadway, New York, New York 10018.
Phone: (212) 966-4320.

Huntington's Chorea Foundation (*Wills Foundation*)
P.O. Box 66704, Houston, Texas 77006.
Phone: (713) 965-9043.

Association to Combat Huntington's Chorea (*COMBAT*)
Lyndhurst Lower Hampton Rd., Sunbury-on-Thames,
Middlesex TW16 5PR, England.
Phone: 01-979-5055.

Huntington Society of Canada
Box 533, Cambridge [Galt], Ontario, Canada, N1R 5T8.
Phone: (519) 622-1002.

Australian Huntington's Disease Association
c/o Department of Psychiatry, University of Melbourne,
Clinical Sciences Building, Royal Melbourne Hospital,
Victoria, Australia 3050.

Vereniging van Huntington
Pa Verkuyllaan 30, 1171 EE Badhoevedorp,
The Netherlands.
Phone: 02960-2921.

Huntington Liga Belgie
Krijkelberg 1, B-3043 Bierbeek, Belgium.

Association Huntington de France
13, rue du 11 novembre, 59650 Villeneuve d'Asoq,
France.

Notes

CHAPTER 1: HUNTINGTON'S DISEASE: WHAT IS IT?

1 The Ian Miller family is fictional. However, this account is based on a composite of real experiences documented in public testimony before the United States Commission for the Control of Huntington's Disease and Its Consequences. See the commission's *Report*, vol. 4.3 (Bethesda, Md.: National Institutes of Health, 1977), pp. 28–32, 505–8, 530–31.

2 G. Huntington, "On chorea," *The Medical and Surgical Reporter* 26 (1872): 317–21. See also D. L. Stevens, "The history of Huntington's chorea," *Journal of the Royal College of Physicians of London* 6 (1972): 271–82; K. W. G. Heathfield, "Huntington's chorea: a centenary review," *Postgraduate Medical Journal* 49 (1973): 32.

3 Huntington's disease (Huntington's chorea), United States Department of Health, Education and Welfare, National Institutes of Health, pub. 76–49 (1976): 12.

4 An excellent general introduction to the science of medical genetics is W. L. Nyhan's *The Hereditary Factor: Genes, Chromosomes, and You* (New York: Grosset and Dunlap, 1976).

5 I. Shoulson and T. N. Chase, "Huntington's disease," *Annual Review of Medicine* 26 (1975): 419–26.

6 I. Shoulson, "Clinical care of the patient and family with Huntington's disease," in *Report: Commission for the Control of Huntington's Disease*, vol. 2, pp. 421–42.

7 W. E. James et al., "Early signs of Huntington's chorea," *Diseases of the Nervous System* 30 (1969): 556–59.

8 Shoulson and Chase, "Huntington's disease," p. 419.

9 R. W. Wells, "Huntington's chorea: seeing beyond the disease," *The American Journal of Nursing* 72 (1972): 954–56.

10 H. L. Klawans and M. M. Cohen, "Diseases of the extrapyramidal system," *Disease-a-Month* (1970): 44–52.

11 *Report: Commission for the Control of Huntington's Disease*, vol. 1, pp. 4, 51–53, 55–63, 85–87.
12 Ibid., vol. 4.3, pp. 562–67.
13 Ibid., pp. 512–13.
14 Ibid., vol. 1, p. 89; I. O. Palmer, "Huntington's chorea," *Nursing Times* 69 (1973): 1015–20.
15 N. S. Wexler, "Genetic 'Russian roulette': the experience of being 'at risk' for Huntington's disease," in S. Kessler, ed., *Genetic Counseling: Psychological Dimensions* (New York: Academic Press, 1979): 397–420.
16 For the address of this and similar organizations in other countries, see appendix 2.

CHAPTER 2: HUNTINGTON'S DISEASE: WHAT CAUSES IT?

1 M. W. Strickberger, *Genetics*, 2nd ed. (New York: Macmillan, 1976), p. 3; W. L. Nyhan, *The Heredity Factor: Genes, Chromosomes, and You* (New York: Grosset and Dunlap, 1976), p. 13; A. Milunsky, *Know Your Genes* (Boston: Houghton Mifflin, 1977), p. 49.
2 J. Fast, *Blueprint for Life: The Story of Modern Genetics* (New York: St. Martin's Press, 1964), p. 83.
3 Milunsky, *Know Your Genes*, p. 50.
4 V. M. Riccardi, *The Genetic Approach to Human Disease* (New York: Oxford University Press, 1977), p. 13.
5 V. A. McKusick, *Human Genetics*, 2nd ed. (Englewood Cliffs, N.J.: Prentice-Hall, 1969), pp. 21–25.
6 Milunsky, *Know Your Genes*, pp. 22, 163–83. At age thirty-five the risk is about one in 100. By age forty-five, it is one in forty. See Riccardi, *The Genetic Approach to Human Disease*, p. 5.
7 Milunsky, *Know Your Genes*, p. 32; D. M. Bonner and S. E. Mills, *Heredity* (Englewood Cliffs, N.J.: Prentice-Hall, 1964), p. 95.
8 J. J. Nora and F. C. Fraser, *Medical Genetics: Principles and Practice* (Philadelphia: Lea and Febiger, 1974), pp. 57–62; Milunsky, *Know Your Genes*, p. 34.
9 Milunsky, *Know Your Genes*, pp. 20, 163–64.
10 Nyhan, *The Heredity Factor*, pp. 23–24.
11 A. E. H. Emery, *Elements of Medical Genetics*, 4th ed. (Berkeley: University of California Press, 1975), pp. 100–101.
12 Nyhan, *The Heredity Factor*, pp. 29–30, 154–56.
13 Ibid., p. 17.
14 Ibid., pp. 15–20.
15 Ibid., pp. 217–19. For an explanation of terms, see glossary.

16   Ibid., pp. 223–27. The cost of screening is about $3–4 per child, or perhaps $8–10 million annually in the United States. One untreated PKU child will cost society at least $250,000, not including lost productivity and earning capacity. For every dollar invested in PKU detection, Nyhan concludes, society saves at least five dollars.

17   Ibid., p. 219.

18   Emery, *Elements of Medical Genetics*, pp. 97–99.

19   *Huntington's Chorea: A Booklet for the Families and Friends of Patients with the Disease* (London: Central Council for the Disabled, n.d.), p. 4.

20   C. F. Stevens, "The neuron," *Scientific American* 241.3 (September 1979): 49–59; W. R. Russell, *Explaining the Brain* (London: Oxford University Press, 1975), p. 108.

21   A. J. Dunn and S. C. Bondy, *Functional Chemistry of the Brain* (Flushing, N.Y.: Spectrum, 1974), pp. 6–8; T. J. Teyler, *A Primer of Psychobiology: Brain and Behavior* (San Francisco: W. H. Freeman and Co., 1975), pp. 30–31.

22   H. L. Klawans et al., "Toward an understanding of the pathophysiology of Huntington's chorea," *Confinia Neurologica* 33(1971): 297.

23   G. K. Klintworth, "Huntington's chorea: morphologic contributions of a century," in A. Barbeau et al., eds., *Advances in Neurology*, vol. 1, *Huntington's Chorea, 1872–1972* (New York: Raven Press, 1973), pp. 353–68.

24   T. L. Perry et al., "Huntington's chorea: deficiency of gamma-aminobutyric acid in brain," *New England Journal of Medicine* 288 (1973): 337–42.

25   E. D. Bird et al., "Reduced glutamic-acid-decarboxylase activity in Huntington's chorea," *Lancet* 1.812 (1973): 1090–92. See also P. L. McGeer et al., "Choline acetylase and glutamic acid decarboxylase in Huntington's chorea: a preliminary study," *Neurology* 23 (1973): 912–17.

26   "The cruelest killer," *Newsweek* (27 September 1976); "Hope for a rare disease," *U.S. News & World Report* (18 October 1976); "Little-known disease," *Family Health* (May 1977).

27   T. L. Perry et al., "Isoniazid therapy for Huntington's disease," in T. N. Chase et al., eds., *Advances in Neurology*, vol. 23, *Huntington's Disease* (New York: Raven Press, 1979), p. 785.

28   G. W. Bruyn, "Huntington's chorea: historical, clinical and laboratory synopsis," in P. J. Vinken and G. W. Bruyn, *Handbook of Clinical Neurology*, vol. 6, *Diseases of the Basal Ganglia* (Amsterdam: North-Holland Publishing Co., 1968), p. 342.

29   E. G. S. Spokes, "Dopamine in Huntington's disease: a study of

postmortem brain tissue," in T. N. Chase et al., eds., *Advances in Neurology*, vol. 23, *Huntington's Disease* (New York: Raven Press, 1979), pp. 481–82.

30 E. D. Bird and L. L. Iversen, "Huntington's chorea: post-mortem measurement of glutamic acid decarboxylase, choline acetyltransferase and dopamine in basal ganglia," *Brain* 97 (1974): 457–72.

31 J. S. Gale et al., "Human brain substance P: distribution in controls and Huntington's chorea," *Journal of Neurochemistry* 30 (1978): 633–34.

32 E. G. S. Spokes, "Neurochemical alterations in Huntington's chorea: a study of post-mortem brain tissue," *Brain* 103 (1980): 179–210.

33 A. Barbeau, "Update on the biochemistry of Huntington's disease," in Chase, *Advances in Neurology*, vol. 23, *Huntington's Disease*, pp. 456–57. See also, in the same volume, D. A. Butterfield and W. R. Markesbery, "Erythrocyte membrane alterations in Huntington's disease," pp. 397–408, and S. A. Appel, "Membrane defects in Huntington's disease," pp. 387–96.

34 These questions are examined more fully in chapter 9.

CHAPTER 3: MEETING THE CHALLENGE OF LIVING "AT RISK" FOR HUNTINGTON'S DISEASE

1 B. Linnen, "Marjorie Guthrie sings out against cause of Woody's death," *Minnesota Daily*, 14 October 1977.

2 N. S. Wexler, "Genetic 'Russian Roulette': the experience of being 'at risk' for Huntington's disease," in S. Kessler, ed., *Genetic Counseling: Psychological Dimensions* (New York: Academic Press, 1979), p. 402.

3 *Report: Commission for the Control of Huntington's Disease and Its Consequences*, vol. 1 (Bethesda, Md.: National Institutes of Health, 1977), p. 2.

4 Wexler, "Genetic 'Russian Roulette,' " p. 398.

5 Ibid., p. 418. The quotation at the beginning of this chapter reflects the worry and misery caused by the habit of symptom watching.

6 Wexler, "Genetic 'Russian Roulette,' " p. 419.

7 Ibid., p. 410.

8 L. E. Nee and a patient, "Experiences of a Huntington's disease patient," *Nursing Care* (1976).

9 Wexler, "Genetic 'Russian Roulette,' " p. 399.

10 Ibid., p. 409.

11 Ibid., pp. 408–9.

12 B. Teltscher and B. Davies, "Medical and social problems of Huntington's disease," *Medical Journal of Australia* 1 (1972): 307–8.

13 E. Kübler-Ross, *On Death and Dying* (New York: Macmillan, 1969), chapters 1–8.

14 See articles in *Huntington's (Chorea) Disease: Handbook for Health Professionals* (New York: Committee to Combat Huntington's Disease, 1974).

15 Wexler, "Genetic 'Russian Roulette,'" p. 417.

16 V. E. Frankl, *Man's Search for Meaning: An Introduction to Logotherapy* (London: Hodder and Stoughton, 1964), pp. 110–17.

CHAPTER 4: GENETIC COUNSELING

1 S. C. Reed, "A short history of genetic counseling," *Social Biology* 21 (1974): 334–35; I. H. Porter, "Evolution of genetic counseling in America," in H. A. Lubs and F. de la Cruz, eds., *Genetic Counseling* (New York: Raven Press, 1977), pp. 17–29.

2 F. C. Fraser, "Genetic counseling," *American Journal of Human Genetics* 26 (1974): 637. See also "Genetic counseling: report of an ad hoc committee of the American Society of Human Genetics," *American Journal of Human Genetics* 27 (1975): 240–42.

3 For comparison, see C. J. Epstein, "A position paper on position papers on the organization of genetic counseling," in Lubs and de la Cruz, *Genetic Counseling*, pp. 333–36.

4 V. A. McKusick, *Mendelian Inheritance in Man: Catalogs of Autosomal Dominant, Autosomal Recessive, and X-Linked Phenotypes*, 4th ed. (Baltimore: Johns Hopkins Press, 1975): pp. 114–15.

5 M. Guthrie, "Consumer viewpoint," in Lubs and de la Cruz, *Genetic Counseling*, pp. 562–63.

6 Personal letter to the author, February 1979.

7 J. R. Whittier, "Management of Huntington's chorea: the disease, those affected, and those otherwise involved," in A. Barbeau et al., eds., *Advances in Neurology*, vol. 1, *Huntington's Chorea, 1872–1972* (New York: Raven Press, 1973), p. 747.

8 Guthrie, "Consumer viewpoint," p. 561.

9 F. Hecht and L. B. Holmes, "What we don't know about genetic counseling," *New England Journal of Medicine* 287 (1972): 464–65.

10 V. A. McKusick and R. Claiborne, *Medical Genetics* (New York: H.P. Publishing Co., 1973), p. 221.

11 Ibid.; see also F. C. Fraser, "Genetic counseling," *Hospital Practice* 6 (1971): 49.

12 R. D. Bell, "Huntington's chorea" (paper presented at the Hunting-

ton's Disease Symposium, The University of Texas Health Science Center at San Antonio, 1979).

13 H. T. Lynch, *Dynamic Genetic Counseling for Clinicians* (Springfield, Ill.: C. C. Thomas, 1969), pp. 16–17.

14 Ibid., p. 36.

15 J. S. Pearson, "Family support and counseling in Huntington's disease," *Psychiatric Forum* (Fall 1973): 48.

16 D. C. Wallace to the author, 25 January 1979.

17 C. O. Leonard et al., "Genetic counseling: a consumers' view," *New England Journal of Medicine* 287 (1972): 433, 437. For a discussion of other studies, see M. E. Shaw, "Review of published studies of genetic counseling: a critique," in Lubs and de la Cruz, *Genetic Counseling*, pp. 38–41.

18 E. A. Murphy, "Probabilities in genetic counseling," in D. Bergsma, ed., "Contemporary genetic counseling," *Birth Defects* 9 (1973): 21.

19 Fraser, "Genetic counseling," *American Journal of Human Genetics*, p. 650.

20 A. Falek, "Use of the coping process to achieve psychological homeostasis in genetic counseling," in Lubs and de la Cruz, *Genetic Counseling*, p. 182.

21 J. R. Sorenson and A. J. Culbert, "Genetic counselors and counseling orientations—unexamined topics in evaluation," in Lubs and de la Cruz, *Genetic Counseling*, pp. 140–51; F. C. Fraser, "Degree of directiveness," in Lubs and de la Cruz, *Genetic Counseling*, pp. 579–81.

22 Fraser, "Genetic counseling," *American Journal of Human Genetics*, p. 649.

23 Pearson, "Family support and counseling in Huntington's disease," pp. 46–50.

24 See A. Milunsky's comments in a discussion in Lubs and de la Cruz, *Genetic Counseling*, p. 580.

25 Lynch, *Dynamic Genetic Counseling for Clinicians*, p. 26.

26 Ibid., p. 21.

27 D. C. Wallace to the author, 21 April 1979.

28 McKusick and Claiborne, *Medical Genetics*, p. 247.

29 C. R. MacKay and J. M. Shea, "Ethical considerations in research on Huntington's disease," *Clinical Research* 25 (1977): 244.

30 Fraser, "Genetic counseling," *American Journal of Human Genetics*, p. 649.

31 Ibid., p. 650.

32 Guthrie, "Consumer viewpoint," p. 564.

33 Pearson, "Family support and counseling in Huntington's disease," p. 49.

34 See chapter 6.

35 "An expanded role for genetic counseling," in *Report: Commission for the Control of Huntington's Disease and Its Consequences*, vol. 2 (Bethesda, Md.: National Institutes of Health, 1977), p. 352.

36 Lynch, *Dynamic Genetic Counseling for Clinicians*, p. 198.

37 V. A. McKusick, "Editorial: family-oriented follow-up," *Journal of Chronic Diseases* 22 (1969): 1–7.

38 W. W. Sly, "What is genetic counseling?" in Bergsma, "Contemporary genetic counseling," pp. 11–12.

39 D. C. Wallace to the author, 21 April 1979.

CHAPTER 5: MANAGEMENT

1 The name Suzan Smith is fictional, but the case is based on actual experiences. See *Report: Commission for the Control of Huntington's Disease and Its Consequences*, vol. 2 (Bethesda, Md.: National Institutes of Health, 1977), pp. 541, 571–73.

2 Ibid., vol. 4, parts 1–6.

3 M. Pines, "What people were telling the commission," in *Report: Commission for the Control of Huntington's Disease*, vol. 2, pp. 571–81.

4 S. L. Ryder, "Design for care," in *Report: Commission for the Control of Huntington's Disease*, vol. 2, pp. 540–41.

5 *Report: Commission for the Control of Huntington's Disease*, vol. 1, pp. 65–66.

6 H. L. Klawans and M. M. Cohen, "Diseases of the extrapyramidal system," *Disease-a-Month* (1970): pp. 49–50.

7 R. R. Howell, "Genetic disease: the present status of treatment," in V. A. McKusick and R. Claiborne, *Medical Genetics* (New York: H.P. Publishing Co., 1973), p. 271.

8 "Secrets of the human cell," *Newsweek* 94 (international ed., 20 August 1979): 42.

9 S. Fahn, "Treatment of choreic movements with perphenazine," in A. Barbeau et al., eds., *Advances in Neurology*, vol. 1, *Huntington's Chorea, 1872–1972* (New York: Raven Press, 1973), p. 755.

10 *Gould Medical Dictionary*, 3rd ed. (New York: McGraw-Hill, 1972), p. 1208.

11 Drugs which increase dopamine transmission in the brain tend to worsen chorea, whereas drugs which deplete dopamine tend to suppress the involuntary muscle movements in HD. Shoulson has summarized the function of various drugs with respect to dopamine: " . . . drugs which block dopaminergic function either by inhibiting dopamine synthesis (alpha-menthylparatyrosine), intraneuronal

storage (resperine or tetrabenazine) or postsynaptic interactions (phenothiazines or butyrophoenone derivatives) are modestly effective in suppressing the motor symptoms of HD." See I. Shoulson, "Huntington's disease," *Annual Review of Medicine* 26 (1975): 422. See also S. J. Enna, "Neurobiology and pharmacology of Huntington's disease," *Life Sciences* 20 (1977): 208.

12 I. Shoulson et al., "Clinical care of the patient and family with Huntington's disease" (New York: Committee to Combat Huntington's Disease, 1978), p. 10.

13 T. L. Perry to the author, 9 April 1980.

14 K. Dewhurst et al., "Socio-psychiatric consequences of Huntington's disease," *British Journal of Psychiatry* 116 (1970): 255–58.

15 Shoulson, "Huntington's disease," p. 424.

16 J. Whittier et al., "Effect of imipramine (tofrānil) on depression and hyperkinesia in Huntington's disease," *American Journal of Psychiatry* 118 (1961): 79.

17 S. E. Folstein et al., "Psychiatric syndromes in Huntington's disease," in T. N. Chase et al., eds., *Advances in Neurology*, vol. 23, *Huntington's Disease* (New York: Raven Press, 1979), pp. 286–87.

18 Shoulson, "Huntington's disease," p. 424.

19 Whittier, "Effect of imipramine," p. 79.

20 E. Miller, "The social work component in community-based action on behalf of victims of Huntington's disease," *Social Work in Health Care* 2 (1976): 27–30.

21 C. Binswanger, "Physical therapy used to extend the creative functional lives of patients with Huntington's disease," in *Huntington's (Chorea) Disease: Handbook for Health Professionals*, condensed ed. (New York: Committee to Combat Huntington's Disease, 1974), p. 17.

22 L. E. Nee and a patient, "Experiences of a Huntington's disease patient" (New York: Committee to Combat Huntington's Disease, n.d.), p. 4.

23 M. Swiatek, "Recreation therapy," in *Huntington's (Chorea) Disease: Handbook for Health Professionals*, p. 7.

24 D. Erdomez, "Music therapy in Huntington's disease" (paper delivered at the First Australian Huntington's Disease Conference, Balwyn, Victoria, 5 November 1979).

25 P. H. Borgelt and T. F. Linde, "A creative attack on Huntington's chorea (occupational therapy)," in *Huntington's (Chorea) Disease: Handbook for Health Professionals*, pp. 15–16.

26 See, for example, the two cases reported in B. Teltscher and B. Davies, "Medical and social problems of Huntington's disease," *The Medical Journal of Australia* 1 (1972): 309–10.

27 It is instructive that most of the authors cited above as experts in the direct care of HD patients are women.

28 J. W. Free and C. McPhillips, "Huntington's disease: how to solve its unique care problems," *RN* 40 (1977): 44.

29 J. Kelly, "Nursing care study. Huntington's chorea: a mother shunned by her family," *Nursing Mirror* 148 (1979): 45–46.

30 "Guidelines for Centers Without Walls," in *Report: Commission for the Control of Huntington's Disease*, vol. 2, pp. 213–15.
    In July, 1980, NINCDS made two five-year grants totalling more than $5 million for the establishment of Centers Without Walls in Baltimore and Boston. These centers will be devoted to research on Huntington's disease and other neurological disorders characterized by brain degeneration and abnormal body movements.

CHAPTER 6: PREDICTIVE TESTING AND EARLY DETECTION

1 A. Barbeau, "Progress in understanding Huntington's chorea," *Canadian Journal of Neurological Sciences* 2 (1975): 83.

2 D. N. Propert, "Presymptomatic detection of Huntington's disease," *Medical Journal of Australia* 1 (1980): 609; T. M. Powledge and J. Fletcher, "Guidelines for the ethical, social and legal issues in prenatal diagnosis," *New England Journal of Medicine* 300 (1979): 168–72; "Ethical guidelines for the development and use of a presymptomatic test," in *Report: Commission for the Control of Huntington's Disease and Its Consequences*, vol. 2 (Bethesda, Md.: National Institutes of Health, 1977), pp. 333–41.

3 R. M. Goodman et al., "Thoughts on the early detection of Huntington's chorea," in A. Barbeau et al., eds., *Advances in Neurology*, vol. 1, *Huntington's Chorea, 1872–1972* (New York: Raven Press, 1973), p. 278.

4 Ibid., pp. 273–74.

5 W. L. Nyhan, *The Heredity Factor: Genes, Chromosomes, and You* (New York: Grosset and Dunlap, 1976), p. 157.

6 Ibid., p. 162.

7 Propert, "Presymptomatic detection of Huntington's disease," p. 610. See also J. E. Oliver, "Abortion and Huntington's chorea" (letter), *British Medical Journal* 1.595 (1968): 576–77.

8 Nyhan, *The Heredity Factor*, pp. 163–64.

9 L. K. Altman, "Birth-defect suits worry doctors," *New York Times*, 30 January 1979.

10 Ibid.

11 Powledge and Fletcher, "Guidelines for the ethical, social and legal issues in prenatal diagnosis," p. 170.

12 R. M. Patterson et al., "The prediction of Huntington's chorea: an electroencephalographic and genetic study," *American Journal of Psychiatry* 104 (1948): 786–97; J. H. Chandler, "EEG in prediction of Huntington's chorea: an eighteen year follow-up," *Electroencephalography and Clinical Neurophysiology* 21 (1966): 79–80; D. F. Scott et al., "The EEG in Huntington's chorea: a clinical and neuropathological study," *Journal of Neurology, Neurosurgery and Psychiatry* 35 (1972): 97–102.

13 I. Shoulson and T. N. Chase, "Huntington's disease," *Annual Review of Medicine* 26 (1975): 421; H. C. Klawans et al., "Predictive test for Huntington's chorea," *Lancet* 2.684 (1970): 1185–86.

14 "Predictive tests in Huntington's chorea," *British Medical Journal* 1.6112 (1978): 528–29.

15 H. L. Klawans et al., "Levodopa and presymptomatic detection of Huntington's disease—eight-year follow-up," *New England Journal of Medicine* 302 (1980): 1090; H. L. Klawans et al., "The use of L-DOPA in the presymptomatic detection of Huntington's chorea," in Barbeau, *Advances in Neurology*, vol. 1, *Huntington's Chorea, 1872–1972*, pp. 295–300; K. W. G. Heathfield, "Huntington's chorea: a centenary review," *Postgraduate Medical Journal* 49 (1973): 38.

16 S. Cederbaum, "Tests for Huntington's chorea," *New England Journal of Medicine* 284 (1971): 1045.

17 "Report of the work group on molecular genetics, virology, immunology, and presymptomatic detection," *Report: Commission for the Control of Huntington's Disease*, vol. 3.1, pp. 40–41.

18 I. S. Cooper, *Living With Chronic Neurologic Disease: A Handbook for Patient and Family* (New York: W. W. Norton and Co., 1976), pp. 119–20.

19 A. N. Neophytides et al., "Computed axial tomography in Huntington's disease and 'at risk' for Huntington's disease," in T. N. Chase et al., eds., *Advances in Neurology*, vol. 23, *Huntington's Disease* (New York: Raven Press, 1979), pp. 185–91; C. F. Terrence et al., "Computed tomography for Huntington's disease," *Neuroradiology* 13 (1977): 173–75.

20 J. A. Lindstrom et al., "Genetic linkage in Huntington's chorea," in Barbeau, *Advances in Neurology*, vol. 1, *Huntington's Chorea, 1872–1972*, pp. 203–8.

21 Propert, "Presymptomatic detection of Huntington's disease," pp. 611–12.

22 D. L. Stevens, "Tests for Huntington's chorea," *New England Journal of Medicine* 285 (1971): 413–14.

23   E. Rothstein, "Huntington's chorea: optimistic view," *New England Journal of Medicine* 285 (1971): 751.

24   R. Stern and R. Eldridge, "Attitudes of patients and their relatives to Huntington's disease," *Journal of Medical Genetics* 12 (1975): 217–23; B. Teltscher and S. Polgar, "Predictive test and Huntington's disease: attitudes of 'at risk' persons to such a test" (paper delivered at the First Australian Huntington's Disease Conference, Balwyn, Victoria, 2–5 November 1979). Teltscher and Polgar found that 88 percent of their respondents who were at risk for the disease felt that persons at risk and considering having children should have a predictive test if one became available.

25   S. Fahn, "Workshop report on research commission on Huntington's chorea of the World Federation of Neurology, Leiden, The Netherlands, 18–21 September 1977," copy supplied by the Committee to Combat Huntington's Disease.

CHAPTER 7: THE WESTPHAL VARIANT AND JUVENILE HUNTINGTON'S DISEASE

1   G. W. Bruyn, "Huntington's chorea: historical, clinical and laboratory synopsis," in P. J. Vinken and G. W. Bruyn, eds., *Handbook of Clinical Neurology*, vol. 6, *Diseases of the Basal Ganglia* (Amsterdam: North-Holland Publishing Co., 1968), p. 323.

2   D. N. Propert, "Genetic markers in the blood of healthy subjects and patients with various mental disorders," (Ph.D. thesis, University of Melbourne, 1977), pp. 416–17.

3   Bruyn, "Huntington's chorea: historical, clinical and laboratory synopsis," pp. 323–24.

4   D. L. Stevens, "The classification of variants of Huntington's chorea," in A. Barbeau et al., eds., *Advances in Neurology*, vol. 1, *Huntington's Chorea, 1872–1972* (New York: Raven Press, 1973), p. 61.

5   Ibid., p. 62.

6   M. T. Bird and G. W. Paulson, "The rigid form of Huntington's chorea," *Neurology* 21 (1971): 271–72.

7   J. B. Bittenbender and F. A. Quadfasel, "Rigid and akinetic forms of Huntington's chorea," *Archives of Neurology* 7 (1962): 275–78; C. J. Brackenridge, "Relation of type of initial symptoms and line of transmission to ages at onset and death in Huntington's disease," *Clinical Genetics* 2 (1971): 287–97.

8   P. Hansotia et al., "Juvenile Huntington's chorea," *Neurology* 18 (1968): 217–18.

9   Ibid., pp. 221, 224.

10   K. W. G. Heathfield, "Huntington's chorea: a centenary review," *Postgraduate Medical Journal*, 49 (1973): 35.

11   Bruyn, "Huntington's chorea: historical, clinical and laboratory synopsis," pp. 323–29.

12   Ibid., p. 329.

13   C. J. Brackenridge, "Relation of parental age to rigidity in Huntington's disease," *Journal of Medical Genetics* 11 (1974): 136–40.

14   Bruyn, "Huntington's chorea: historical, clinical and laboratory synopsis," pp. 316, 323.

15   Ibid., pp. 316–23. See also G. W. Bruyn, "Clinical variants and differential diagnosis," in Barbeau, *Advances in Neurology*, vol. 1, *Huntington's Chorea, 1872–1972*, pp. 51–56; C. Korenyi and J. R. Whittier, "The juvenile form of Huntington's chorea: its prevalence and other observations," in Barbeau, *Advances in Neurology*, vol. 1, *Huntington's Chorea, 1872–1972*, pp. 75–77; and G. A. Jervis, "Huntington's chorea in childhood," *Archives of Neurology* 9 (1963):244–57.

16   Bruyn, "Huntington's chorea: historical, clinical and laboratory synopsis," p. 322.

17   K. E. Dewhurst and J. E. Oliver, "Huntington's disease of young people," *European Neurology* 3 (1970): 278–89. See also J. E. Oliver and K. E. Dewhurst, "Childhood and adolescent forms of Huntington's disease," *Journal of Neurology, Neurosurgery and Psychiatry* 32 (1969): 455–59.

18   J. B. Green et al., "Epilepsy in Huntington's chorea: clinical and neurophysiological studies," in Barbeau, *Advances in Neurology*, vol. 1, *Huntington's Chorea, 1872–1972*, pp. 105–13.

19   R. K. Byers and J. A. Dodge, "Huntington's chorea in children: report of four cases," *Neurology* 17 (1967): 587–96.

20   Ibid., pp. 590–91.

21   A. Barbeau, "Parental ascent in the juvenile form of Huntington's chorea," *Lancet* 2.679 (1970): 937.

22   Propert, "Genetic markers in the blood of healthy subjects and patients with various mental disorders," pp. 420–21.

23   M. B. Jones, "Fertility and age of onset in Huntington's chorea," in Barbeau, *Advances in Neurology*, vol. 1, *Huntington's Chorea, 1872–1972*, p. 174.

24   Propert, "Genetic markers," p. 421.

25   E. D. Bird et al., "A sex-related factor in the inheritance of Huntington's chorea," *Annals of Human Genetics* 37 (1974): 255–60; M. Vegter-Van Der Vlis et al., "Ages of death of children with

Huntington's chorea and of their affected parents," *Annals of Human Genetics* 39 (1976):329–34.

26   C. J. Brackenridge and B. Teltscher, "Estimation of the age at onset of Huntington's disease from factors associated with the affected parent," *Journal of Medical Genetics* 12 (1975):64–69.

27   Oliver and Dewhurst, "Childhood and adolescent forms of Huntington's disease," p. 458.

28   K. E. Dewhurst et al., "Socio-psychiatric consequences of Huntington's disease," *British Journal of Psychiatry* 116 (1970): 255–58.

29   J. E. Oliver, "Huntington's chorea in Northamptonshire," *British Journal of Psychiatry* 116 (1970): 241–53.

30   D. C. Wallace, "Huntington's chorea in Queensland: a not uncommon disease," *The Medical Journal of Australia* 1 (1972): 302.

31   Ibid.

32   Personal testimony in *Report: Commission for the Control of Huntington's Disease and Its Consequences*, vol. 4.3, (Bethesda, Md.: National Institutes of Health, 1977), pp. 447–52.

33   I. S. Cooper, *Living With Chronic Neurologic Disease: A Handbook for Patient and Family* (New York: W. W. Norton and Co., 1976), p. 39.

34   Ibid., p. 36.

35   D. Maddison and B. Raphael, "Social and psychological consequences of chronic disease in childhood," *Medical Journal of Australia* 2.3 (1971): 1265.

36   Ibid.

37   Cooper, *Living With Chronic Neurologic Disease*, pp. 69–71.

38   Ibid., pp. 23, 69–71.

39   Ibid., pp. 23, 71.

CHAPTER 8: SOCIAL PROBLEMS

1   *Report: Commission for the Control of Huntington's Disease and Its Consequences*, vol. 3.2, (Bethesda, Md.: National Institutes of Health, 1977), p. 272.

2   Ibid., vol. 4.4, pp. 239–40.

3   B. Teltscher and B. Davies, "Medical and social problems of Huntington's disease," *Medical Journal of Australia* 1 (1972): 307–10; see also the public testimony in *Report: Commission for the Control of Huntington's Disease*, vol. 4.6, pp. 338–39, 511–12, 516–17, passim.

4   Ibid., p. 620.

5   I. S. Cooper, *Living With Chronic Neurologic Disease: A Handbook*

for Patient and Family (New York: W. W. Norton and Co., 1976), p. 49.

6   Ibid., p. 51.
7   Report: Commission for the Control of Huntington's Disease, vol. 4.4, p. 361.
8   Ibid., vol. 4.6, p. 359.
9   Ibid., p. 387.
10 Ibid., vol. 2, pp. 238–40.
11 Ibid., p. 242.
12 Ibid., p. 247.
13 There is some interesting work being done in this area. See, for example, L. Walters, "Human in vitro fertilization: a review of the ethical literature," The Hastings Center Report 9 (1979): 23–43; and J. Fletcher, The Ethics of Genetic Control: Ending Reproductive Roulette (Garden City, N.Y.: Anchor Press, 1974), p. 165.
14 Report: Commission for the Control of Huntington's Disease, vol. 2, pp. 253–83.

CHAPTER 9: RESEARCH PROSPECTS

1   Report: Commission for the Control of Huntington's Disease and Its Consequences, vol. 1 (Bethesda, Md.: National Institutes of Health, 1977), pp. 15–16.
2   T. N. Chase et al., eds., Advances in Neurology, vol. 23, Huntington's Disease (New York: Raven Press, 1979).
3   L. N. Went and W. S. Volkers, "Genetic linkage," in Chase, Advances in Neurology, vol. 23, Huntington's Disease, p. 37.
4   Report: Commission for the Control of Huntington's Disease, vol. 2, p. 13.
5   L. L. Iversen, "The chemistry of the brain," Scientific American 241.3 (September 1979): 118.
6   T. Caraceni et al., "Biochemical aspects of Huntington's chorea," Journal of Neurology, Neurosurgery and Psychiatry 40 (1977): 581–87; A. Barbeau, "Update on the biochemistry of Huntington's chorea," in Chase, Advances in Neurology, vol. 23, Huntington's Disease, pp. 449–61.
7   T. L. Perry et al., "Huntington's chorea: deficiency of gamma-aminobutyric acid in brain," New England Journal of Medicine 288 (1973): 337–42; S. J. Enna et al., "Huntington's chorea: changes in neurotransmitter receptors in the brain," New England Journal of Medicine 294 (1976): 1305–9. The blood-brain barrier is the functional barrier between the brain capillaries and the brain tissue which allows some substances from the blood to enter the brain

rapidly while other substances either enter slowly or not at all.

8   A. Barbeau, "GABA and Huntington's chorea" (letter), *Lancet* 2.844 (1973): 1499–1500; T. L. Perry et al., "Amino acids in plasma, cerebrospinal fluid and brain of patients with Huntington's chorea," in Barbeau et al., eds., *Advances in Neurology*, vol. 1, *Huntington's Chorea, 1872–1972*, pp. 616–17.

9   W. L. Nyhan, *The Heredity Factor: Genes, Chromosomes, and You* (New York: Grosset and Dunlap, 1976), p. 241.

10   A. Milunsky, *Know Your Genes* (Boston: Houghton Mifflin, 1977), p. 268.

11   G. Husby et al., "Huntington's disease, antineuronal antibodies, brain antigens, and receptors for IgG in human choroid plexus," in Chase, *Advances in Neurology*, vol. 23, *Huntington's Disease*, pp. 435–42.

12   D. S. Barkley and S. I. Hardiwidjaja, "Temporal immunogenetics, Huntington's disease, and multiple sclerosis," in Chase, *Advances in Neurology*, vol. 23, *Huntington's Disease*, p. 430.

13   Ibid., pp. 431–32.

14   Nyhan, *The Heredity Factor*, pp. 77–81.

15   Milunsky, *Know Your Genes*, p. 251.

16   N. C. Myrianthopoulos, "Huntington's chorea: review article," *Journal of Medical Genetics* 3 (1966): 310.

17   A. Barbeau, "Update on the biochemistry of Huntington's chorea," in Chase, *Advances in Neurology*, vol. 23, *Huntington's Disease*, p. 450.

18   "Secrets of the human cell," *Newsweek* 94 (international ed., 20 August 1979): 43.

19   D. A. Butterfield and W. R. Markesbery, "Erythrocyte membrane alterations in Huntington's disease," in Chase, *Advances in Neurology*, vol. 23, *Huntington's Disease*, pp. 397–408.

20   J. H. Menkes and N. Stein, "Fibroblast cultures in Huntington's disease," *New England Journal of Medicine* 288 (1973): 856–57; I. Goetz et al., "Fibroblasts in Huntington's disease," *New England Journal of Medicine*, 293 (1975): 1225–27.

21   G. W. Bruyn, "Neuropathology of Huntington's disease" (paper delivered at the First Australian Huntington's Disease Conference, Balwyn, Victoria, 2 November 1979).

22   E. D. Bird, "Neuroendocrine changes in Huntington's disease: an overview," in Chase, *Advances in Neurology*, vol. 23, *Huntington's Disease*, pp. 291–97.

23   K. W. G. Heathfield, "Huntington's chorea: a centenary review," *Postgraduate Medical Journal* 49 (1973): 40.

24   E. E. Müller et al., "Dopaminergic drugs on growth hormone and

prolactin secretion in Huntington's disease," in Chase, *Advances in Neurology*, vol. 23, *Huntington's Disease*, pp. 319–34.

25   Bird, "Neuroendocrine changes," pp. 292–93.

26   A. N. Moshell et al., "Radiosensitivity in Huntington's disease: implications for pathogenesis and presymptomatic diagnosis," *Lancet* 1 (1980): 9–11.

27   J. T. Coyle and R. Schwarez, "Lesion of striatal neurons with kainic acid provides a model for Huntington's chorea," *Nature* 263 (1976): 244–46.

28   R. L. Borison and B. I. Diamond, "A new animal model for Huntington's disease," in Chase, *Advances in Neurology*, vol. 23, *Huntington's Disease*, pp. 669–77.

29   E. G. McGeer and P. L. McGeer, "Duplication of biochemical changes of Huntington's chorea by intrastriatal injections of glutamic and kainic acids," *Nature* 263 (1976): 517–18.

30   J. W. Olney and T. de Gubareff, "Glutamate neurotocity and Huntington's chorea," *Nature* 271 (1978): 557–59; G. A. R. Johnston, "Glutamic acid and Huntington's disease" (paper delivered at the First Australian Huntington's Disease Conference, Balwyn, Victoria, 2 November 1979).

31   A. Barbeau, "Quebec cooperative study of Friedreich's Ataxia: design of the investigation," *Canadian Journal of Neurological Sciences* (1976): 271–74.

32   *Report: Commission for the Control of Huntington's Disease*, vol. 1, pp. 101–8.

33   I. S. Cooper, *Living With Chronic Neurologic Disease: A Handbook for Patient and Family* (New York: W. W. Norton and Co., 1976), p. 47.

CHAPTER 10: HISTORY

1   G. Huntington, "Recollections of Huntington's chorea as I saw it at East Hampton, Long Island, during my boyhood," in A. Barbeau et al., eds., *Advances in Neurology*, vol. 1, *Huntington's Chorea, 1872–1972* (New York: Raven Press, 1973), pp. 37–39.

2   G. Huntington, "On chorea," *The Medical and Surgical Reporter* 26 (1872): 317–21; R. N. DeJong, "The history of Huntington's chorea in the United States of America," in Barbeau, *Advances in Neurology*, vol. 1, *Huntington's Chorea, 1872–1972*, pp. 19–27.

3   D. L. Stevens, "The history of Huntington's chorea," *Journal of the Royal College of Physicians of London* 6 (1972): 271.

4   J. Bell, "Huntington's chorea," in R. A. Fisher and L. S. Penrose, eds., *The Treasury of Human Inheritance*, vol. 4 (London: Cam-

bridge University Press, 1948), p. 1; G. W. Bruyn, "Huntington's chorea: historical, clinical and laboratory synopsis," in P. J. Vinken and G. W. Bruyn, eds., *Handbook of Clinical Neurology*, vol. 6, *Diseases of the Basal Ganglia* (Amsterdam: North-Holland Publishing Co., 1968), p. 301.

5 G. W. Paulson, "A neurologist speaks with Huntington's disease families" (New York: National Huntington's Disease Association, n.d.), p. 1.

6 *Report: Commission for the Control of Huntington's Disease and Its Consequences*, vol. 1 (Bethesda, Md.: National Institutes of Health, 1977), p. xvii; J. H. Bjorklund, "HD victims: all is not gloom," *San Francisco Sunday Examiner and Chronicle*, 30 October 1977.

7 J. Bell commenting on the work of Lyon in "Huntington's chorea," in Fisher and Penrose, *The Treasury of Human Inheritance*, p. 4.

8 Ibid., p. 1.

9 G. W. Bruyn, "Huntington's chorea: historical, clinical and laboratory synopsis," in Vinken and Bruyn, *Handbook of Clinical Neurology*, vol. 6, p. 298.

10 J. Elliotson, "St. Vitus' dance," *Lancet* 1 (1832): 161.

11 G. W. Bruyn, "Huntington's chorea: historical, clinical and laboratory synopsis," in Vinken and Bruyn, *Handbook of Clinical Neurology*, vol. 6, p. 298.

12 Quoted in DeJong, "History of Huntington's chorea in the United States of America," in Barbeau, *Advances in Neurology*, vol. 1, *Huntington's Chorea, 1872–1972*, p. 21.

13 See the reprint of Lyon's "Chronic hereditary chorea," from *American Medical Times* (19 December 1863) in Barbeau, *Advances in Neurology*, vol. 1, *Huntington's Chorea, 1872–1972*, pp. 31–32.

14 G. W. Bruyn, "Huntington's chorea: historical, clinical and laboratory synopsis," in Vinken and Bruyn, *Handbook of Clinical Neurology*, vol. 6, p. 299.

15 Stevens, "The history of Huntington's chorea," pp. 274–75.

16 A. H. Sturtevant, *A History of Genetics* (New York: Harper and Row, 1965), pp. 9–29.

17 Stevens, "The history of Huntington's chorea," p. 277.

18 Ibid., pp. 277–78.

19 P. R. Vessie, "On the transmission of Huntington's chorea for 300 years: the Bures family group," *Journal of Nervous and Mental Disorders* 76 (1932): 553–73.

20 M. B. Hans and T. H. Gilmore, "Huntington's chorea and genealogical credibility," *Journal of Nervous and Mental Disease* 148 (1969): 5–13.

21 A. Barbeau et al., "La chorée de Huntingdon chez les Canadiens

Français," *Union Médicale de Canada* 93 (1964): 1178.

22   M. Critchley, "Huntington's chorea in East Anglia," *Journal of State Medicine* 42 (1934): 575. See also Critchley's "Great Britain and the early history of Huntington's chorea," in Barbeau, *Advances in Neurology*, vol. 1, *Huntington's Chorea, 1872–1972*, pp. 12–17.

23   C. R. D. Brothers, "The history and incidence of Huntington's chorea in Tasmania," *Royal Australasian College of Physicians* 4 (1949): 47–50.

24   C. R. D. Brothers and A. W. Meadows, "An investigation of Huntington's chorea in Victoria," *Journal of Mental Science* 101 (1955): 548; N. Parker, "Observations on Huntington's chorea based on a Queensland survey," *Medical Journal of Australia* 1 (1958): 351; B. Teltscher to the author, 3 March 1980.

25   F. Gale and J. H. Bennett, "Huntington's chorea in a South Australian community of aboriginal descent," *Medical Journal of Australia* 2 (1969): 482–84.

26   D. C. Wallace, "Huntington's chorea in Queensland: a not uncommon disease," *Medical Journal of Australia* 1 (1972): 299.

27   J. R. Whittier et al., "Prevalence of Huntington's chorea" (letter), *Journal of the American Medical Association* 226 (1973): 1465–66. See also C. Korenyi and J. R. Whittier, "Huntington's disease (chorea) in New York state: approximate gene prevalence in New York City and on Long Island," *New York State Journal of Medicine* 77 (1977): 44–45.

28   Wallace, "Huntington's chorea in Queensland: a not uncommon disease," p. 300. See also D. C. Wallace and N. Parker, "Huntington's chorea in Queensland: the most recent story," in Barbeau, *Advances in Neurology*, vol. 1, *Huntington's Chorea 1872–1972*, pp. 223–36. For prevalence reports on the disease in Belgium, Japan, Venezuela, and various American states, see pp. 237–69 in the same volume.

29   Wallace, "Huntington's chorea in Queensland: a not uncommon disease," p. 301; J. F. Kurtzke, "Huntington's disease: mortality and morbidity data from outside the United States," in T. N. Chase et al., *Advances in Neurology*, vol. 23, *Huntington's Disease* (New York: Raven Press, 1979), pp. 13–25.

30   Whittier, "Prevalence of Huntington's chorea," p. 1465; R. LL. Lyon, "Huntington's chorea in the Moray Firth area," *British Medical Journal* 5288 (1962): 1301–6.

31   R. Avila-Giron, "Medical and social aspects of Huntington's chorea in the state of Zulia, Venezuela," in Barbeau, *Advances in Neurology*, vol. 1, *Huntington's Chorea, 1872–1972*, pp. 261–66.

32   M. Guthrie, "A personal view of genetic counseling," in Y. E. Hsia et al., eds., *Counseling in Genetics* (New York: Alan R. Liss, Inc., 1979), p. 336.

33   "Decade of progress and hope, 1967–1977." (New York: Committee to Combat Huntington's Disease, 1977), p. 5; *Report: Commission for the Control of Huntington's Disease*, vol. 1, p. 101.

34   See M. Guthrie's transmittal letters to the President of the United States and to the Congress in *Report: Commission for the Control of Huntington's Disease*, vol. 1.

35   M. Wexler to the author, 10 September 1979.

36   W. Hatter (president of the National Huntington's Disease Association) to the author, 17 September 1979.

37   F. Pratt (president of the Wills Foundation) to the author, 10 September and 30 October 1979.

38   M. Jones to the author, 27 September 1979.

39   R. Walker to the author, 21 November 1979.

40   B. Teltscher to the author, 3 March 1980; E. Chiu and B. Teltscher, "Huntington's disease: the establishment of a national register," *Medical Journal of Australia* 2 (1978): 394–96.

41   F. Baro (professor of neuropsychiatry at the Katholieke Universiteit Leuven) to the author, 2 September 1980.

42   "Huntington's international," in Newsletter 17, Association to Combat Huntington's Chorea (September 1979), p. 8.

Glossary

Acetylcholine: A compound in the body which affects muscle action, inhibits heart activity, and influences digestion and dilation of the blood vessels.

Allele: One of two or more alternative forms of a gene.

Alzheimer's disease: Progressive dementia caused by severe damage to certain cells in the brain.

Amino acids: A large group of compounds from which the body synthesizes its proteins.

Amniocentesis: Medical procedure for prenatal screening for a variety of abnormalities. A sample of the fluid in which the embryo is suspended in the uterus is extracted and analyzed.

Antibody: A substance produced by the body in response to a foreign agent, with the specific capacity to create immunity to and neutralize that agent.

Antigen: A substance capable of provoking an immunologic response, such as the production of an antibody specific for that substance.

Astrocyte: A star-shaped cell attached to the blood vessels of the brain and spinal cord.

Ataxia: Incoordination of voluntary muscular action, particularly of the muscle groups used in activities such as walking or reaching for objects.

Ataxia telangiectasia: A recessive genetic disorder characterized by onset of progressive cerebellar ataxia in infancy or childhood.

Athetosis: Involuntary movements characterized by recurrent, slow, worm-like change of position of the fingers, toes, hands, feet, and other parts of the body.

Atrophy: The wasting away of tissues, organs, or the entire body.

Autoimmunity: A condition which results when the body's defense mechanisms fail to recognize normally occurring substances, responding to them as if they were foreign antigens.

Autosomal dominant disease: A disorder caused by the presence of a single defective dominant gene located on a chromosome other than the sex chromosomes. Huntington's disease is an autosomal dominant disorder.

Autosomal inheritance: Transmission of genetic characteristics not related to sex.

Autosomal recessive disease: A disorder caused by the presence of two defective recessive genes located on a chromosome other than the sex chromosomes.

Autosome: A non-sex-determining chromosome.

Basal ganglia: An area of brain tissue located at the base of the cerebrum, primarily influencing motor control; seriously damaged by Huntington's disease.

Biopsy: The removal and examination of tissue from the living body.

Carrier: A person harboring a disease who, though often not exhibiting symptoms, may transmit the disease to others. In genetics, a carrier is an individual whose chromosomes contain the gene for a specific genetic condition.

Cerebral cortex: Gray outer layer of brain tissue, largely responsible for higher mental processes such as thinking, perception, and memory.

Cerebrospinal fluid (CSF): The serum-like fluid that bathes portions of the brain and the cavity of the spinal cord.

Cerebrum: The largest part of the brain, consisting of two halves or hemispheres.

Chorea: Any of the disorders characterized by irregular and involuntary movements of the extremities and the face; common in many neurological disorders, such as Huntington's disease.

Chromosomes: The thread-like bodies in the cell nucleus, composed of linked DNA nucleotides, or genes, responsible for carrying hereditary characteristics from one generation to the next.

Computerized axial tomography (CAT): Computerized technique for making x-ray pictures of portions of the body, usually the head or trunk, to assist in medical diagnosis and analysis.

Cystinosis: An autosomal recessive disease affecting metabolism, in which the amino acid cystine accumulates in body tissues. Prenatal diagnosis is possible.

Cytogenetics: The study of chromosomes.

Dementia: Deterioration or loss of intellectual faculties, reasoning power, memory, and will, caused by organic brain disease; characterized by varying degrees of confusion, disorientation, and stupor.

Deoxyribonucleic acid (DNA): The basic genetic material. Its molecular structure determines the replication of the genetic code and governs the formation of proteins.

Dominant gene: A gene, or DNA sequence, whose expression prevails over those of alternative alleles for a given trait. A child inheriting a dominant gene for brown eyes and a recessive gene for blue eyes will have brown eyes. Huntington's disease is a dominant genetic disorder.

Dopamine: A chemical substance essential to normal nerve cell activity in the brain.

Down's syndrome: A chromosomal disorder resulting from the presence of an extra autosome with chromosome pair 21. Characteristics include retarded growth, flattened skull, slanting eyes, and thickened tongue. Also known as "mongolism."

Dyskinesia: Difficulty in performing voluntary movements.

Electroencephalogram (EEG): A graphic record of the electrical activity of the brain.

Electron spin resonance: An experimental technique for investigating biological structures (such as proteins) by introducing various "labels" (special compounds) into these structures in order to monitor them more precisely; also known as electron paramagnetic resonance spectroscopy.

Encephalitis: Inflammation of the brain.

Encephalopathy: Any disease of the brain.

Endocrinology: The branch of medicine dealing with the internal secretions of the body.

Enzymes: Protein molecules synthesized according to instructions from the DNA code. Enzymes control the rate of all metabolic processes within the body.

Epidemiology: The study of the frequency and distribution of a disease in a community.

Epilepsy: A chronic brain disorder of various causes characterized by recurrent seizures due to excessive electrical discharge by cerebral neurons.

Expressivity: The degree to which a gene is overtly manifested within an individual. Two persons who have the same gene for a genetic disorder may show symptoms of different severity.

Factor VIII: A blood protein essential for clotting. Persons with hemophilia are unable to produce this substance.

Fibroblasts: Large spindle-shaped cells, common in developing tissues and tissues that are under repair.

Friedreich's ataxia: A hereditary spinocerebellar degenerative disease characterized by a loss of muscular coordination.

Gamma-aminobutyric acid (GABA): A substance in the central nervous system which functions to inhibit nerve impulses.

Gaucher's disease: An autosomal recessive degenerative disease of the nervous system whose symptoms include enlargement of the spleen. Prenatal detection is possible.

Gene: A portion of the DNA molecule in the cell chromosome. Genes are responsible for carrying hereditary characteristics from one generation to the next.

Genetic counseling: Counseling specifically dealing with the human problems associated with the occurrence, or risk of occurrence, of a genetic disorder.

Genetic engineering: A field of scientific inquiry that focuses on the prevention or remission of inherited disorders, and other goals, by manipulation of genetic material.

Genetics: The branch of biology that deals with heredity and variation.

Genotype: The hereditary constitution of an organism resulting from its particular combination of genes. A class of individuals having the same genetic constitution.

Glutamic acid: An amino acid. Its presence is necessary for the production of normal hemoglobin, the protein of red blood cells that carries oxygen to body tissues.

Glutamic acid decarboxylase (GAD):   A substance in the brain which is involved in the formation of gamma-aminobutyric acid (GABA).

Glycogen: A substance which is formed from carbohydrates, stored in the liver, and converted into sugar as the body requires.

Grand mal: Generalized seizure.

Hemophilia: A bleeding disorder of sex-linked recessive transmission, in which the body fails to produce a protein required to make the blood clot properly.

Heterozygous: Having dissimilar members in one or more pairs of genes.

Homozygous: Having like members in a given pair of genes.

Hunter's syndrome: An X-linked recessive disease whose symptoms include coarsening of facial features, enlargement of the liver and spleen, and severe mental retardation. Prenatal detection is possible.

Huntington's disease: An autosomal dominant genetic disorder, with onset usually in middle age, characterized by abnormal involuntary movements (chorea), progressive intellectual impairment (dementia), and a spectrum of psychiatric disturbances. The disease is progressive and terminal over a period of ten to twenty years.

Hurler's syndrome: An autosomal recessive disease characterized by misshapen bones, enlarged liver and spleen, poor vision, and mental retardation. Prenatal detection is possible.

Hypothalamus: A part of the brain that regulates many basic body functions, such as body temperature and appetite.

Inhibitory neurotransmitters: Chemical agents which have a restraining effect on the firing of nerve impulses.

In utero: Within the uterus; not yet born; from the Latin, meaning "in the womb."

In vitro: From the Latin, meaning "in glass"; refers to a process or reaction occurring in a culture dish or test tube.

In vivo: From the Latin, meaning "in the living"; refers to a process within, or a study done on, a living organism.

Irradiation: Exposure to radiation.

Kainic acid: A chemical substance used in experiments on animals which destroys some of the same cells in animal brains that are destroyed in human brains by Huntington's disease.

Karyotype: The chromosome complement of an individual. In the normal human being the karyotype consists of twenty-two pairs of autosomes and one pair of sex chromosomes.

Kayser-Fleischer ring: A green ring that appears in the cornea of the eye in patients with Wilson's disease, resulting from an excessive accumulation of copper.

Klinefelter's syndrome: A disorder occurring in males who have an extra X chromosome (XXY).

L-DOPA: Drug used for the treatment of Parkinson's disease.

Metabolism: The process of synthesizing foodstuffs into complex elements and complex substances into simple ones for the production of energy.

Metabolite: Any molecule that is a product of metabolism.

Morphology: A branch of biology that deals with the form and structure of animals and plants; also the branch of pathology that deals with abnormal form and structure of disease tissue.

Multiple sclerosis: A chronic, degenerative neurological disease found chiefly in young adults and characterized by hardening of the tissues of the brain and/or spinal cord. The cause is unknown.

Muscular dystrophy: Inherited progressive wasting of the voluntary muscles of the body. There are many different forms of the disease.

Myoclonic epilepsy: Recurrent irregular spasms of a muscle or groups of muscles varying in intensity and usually without evident alteration of consciousness.

Neuroanatomy: The science of the structure of the nervous system.

Neurobiology: The study of the functions of the brain and the nervous system.

Neurological disorders: Organic diseases of the nervous system.

Neurology: Study of the anatomy, physiology and pathology of the nervous system.

Neurons: Nerve cells.

Neuropathology: The science concerned with the causes and development of diseases of the nervous system.

Neuropharmacology: The study of drugs that produce an effect on nervous tissue.

Neurosis: Psychological or behavioral disorder often characterized by anxiety.

Neurotransmitter: A chemical substance influencing the transmission of nerve impulses.

Niemann-Pick disease: An autosomal recessive disease whose symptoms include enlargement of the spleen and liver and neurological degeneration. Prenatal detection is possible.

Nucleotide: The basic structural unit of nucleic acid. Every nucleotide is composed of a chemically bonded phosphate, a sugar, and one of several nitrogen-containing base molecules.

Parkinson's disease: A progressive nervous disease causing muscular tremors, rigidity of movement, and peculiarities of gait, posture, and facial expression.

Pathogenesis: The origin and development of a disease.

Pathology: The study of the essential nature of diseases and especially of the structural and functional changes produced by them.

Penetrance: The frequency with which a gene produces its specific effect in its carriers in a population. Huntington's disease is said to be "completely penetrant" because, if present, the gene always manifests itself, provided the carrier lives a normal lifespan.

Phenotype: An observable characteristic expressed by a gene or genes in combination; also, a category or group to which an individual may be assigned on the basis of characteristics resulting from both its heredity and its environment.

Phenylketonuria (PKU): An autosomal recessive genetic disease. Absence of an active liver enzyme produces severe mental retardation. Treated by means of a special diet.

Placebo: A preparation, devoid of pharmacological effect, given for psychological effect; a worthless pill given to humor a patient.

Platelets: Small, irregular disk-shaped elements in the blood, vital to the clotting process.

Polydactylism: The condition of having too many fingers or toes.

Pompe syndrome: An autosomal recessive disease in which heart failure results from storage of glycogen in the heart muscle. Prenatal detection is possible.

Presenile dementia: Premature old age, or premature appearance of the infirmities associated with it; especially, any chronic organic brain disorder characterized by premature senility.

Presymptomatic test: Test used for the detection of the existence of a disease before any symptoms appear.

Protein: A major component of all living things; one of a group of complex substances composed of amino acids linked together in large molecules.

Radiomimetic: Capable of producing biological effects similar to those of ionizing radiation.

Recessive trait: A genetic trait produced by the occurrence of two like recessive genes. A recessive gene that occurs together with its dominant allele is never expressed, but gives way to the dominant trait.

Schizophrenia: A severe mental disorder resulting in withdrawal from reality and emotional and intellectual disturbances.

Sex-linked inheritance: Inheritance of traits determined by genes located on the sex chromosomes.

Sickle cell anemia: A recessive genetic disease, especially common among black populations, in which some red blood cells become deformed into sickle shapes, causing blockages in blood vessels.

Sydenham's chorea: An infectious nervous disease occurring in young persons and causing involuntary muscle movements of the face, neck, and limbs.

Syndrome: Any group of symptoms that occur in association with each other.

Tardive dyskinesia: A persistent disorder characterized by excessive muscular activity, occurring after withdrawal from certain drugs.

Tay-Sachs disease: A rare, recessive hereditary disorder causing mental retardation, paralysis, and death in early childhood. The disease is transmitted by a gene common in Ashkenazic Jews. Prenatal detection is possible.

Transferase: Enzymes that catalyze transfer of a chemical group from one molecule to another.

Trisomy 21:   Presence of an extra (third) autosome 21, which produces Down's syndrome.

Turner's syndrome: A disorder caused by the presence in females of only one X chromosome; occurs about once in every 3,500 female births. Persons with this condition typically are short and have underdeveloped ovaries.

Virology: The study of viruses and viral diseases.

Virus: A minute structure, composed of a sheath of protein encasing a core of nucleic acids, which replicates parasitically within the cell of its host. Many hundreds of viruses have been identified; almost all members of the plant and animal kingdoms are vulnerable to viral infections.

Wilson's disease: An autosomal recessive disorder characterized by neurological deterioration, muscular rigidity, garbled speech, and a green ring in the cornea. Symptoms of the disease are caused by an abnormal metabolism of copper, and can be managed with drugs which help to eliminate copper from the body.

X chromosome: A sex-determining factor in ova and approximately one-half of sperm. Ova fertilized by sperm having the X chromosome give rise to female offspring.

Xeroderma pigmentosum: An autosomal recessive genetic disorder involving the skin. Prenatal diagnosis is possible.

Y chromosome: A sex-determining factor in about one-half of the sperm. Ova fertilized by sperm carrying the Y chromosome give rise to male offspring.

Zygote: A fertilized egg that results from the fusion of a sperm and ovum.

Bibliography

Four sources were particularly important in the writing of this book. The first was the ten-volume *Report: Commission for the Control of Huntington's Disease and Its Consequences.* This exhaustive report contains public testimony, technical submissions, and detailed recommendations for a national plan of attack against Huntington's disease and related disorders.

The second source was André Barbeau, Thomas N. Chase, and George W. Paulson, eds., *Advances in Neurology. Volume 1. Huntington's Chorea, 1872–1972* (New York: Raven Press, 1973). The volume is a compilation of the scientific papers which were delivered at the Centennial Symposium on Huntington's Disease in Ohio in 1972.

In November, 1978, the Second International Symposium on Huntington's Disease convened in San Diego, California. Several hundred physicians and scientists from more than a dozen nations attended this forum. Out of the meeting came the third vital source for this book: Thomas N. Chase, Nancy S. Wexler, and André Barbeau, eds., *Advances in Neurology. Volume 23. Huntington's Disease* (New York: Raven Press, 1979). Papers contained in the two volumes of the *Advances in Neurology* series have been cited individually in the notes of this book.

The fourth major source of material was medical and scientific journals. A quick look through *Index Medicus* reveals that there has been an explosion of interest in Huntington's disease research in recent years.

This bibliography is not intended as a comprehensive guide to the literature. The sources listed are those that proved most useful for research on this book. More detailed bibliographies on Huntington's disease are readily available from among these sources.

BIBLIOGRAPHICAL AIDS

Boyes, J. W., et al. *References to Nomenclature and Other Publications in*

Genetics and Cytology (Montreal: International Genetics Foundation, 1973).

Bruyn, G. W., et al. *A Centennial Bibliography of Huntington's Chorea, 1872–1972* (Louvain: Leuven University Press, 1974).

Cumulated Index Medicus (Washington, D.C.: Government Printing Office).

BOOKS

Asimov, I. *The Human Brain: Its Capacities and Functions*. Boston: Houghton Mifflin, 1963.

Asimov, I. *The Genetic Code*. London: John Murray, 1964.

Barbeau, A., et al., eds. *Advances in Neurology*. Vol. 1. *Huntington's Chorea, 1872–1972*. New York: Raven Press, 1973.

Bonner, D. M., and S. E. Mills. *Heredity*. 2nd ed. Englewood Cliffs, N.J.: Prentice-Hall, 1964.

Chase, T. N., et al., eds. *Advances in Neurology*. Vol. 23. *Huntington's Disease*. New York: Raven Press, 1979.

Cooper, I. S. *Living With Chronic Neurologic Disease: A Handbook for Patient and Family*. New York: W. W. Norton and Co., 1976.

Dunkerley, G. B. *A Basic Atlas of the Human Nervous System*. Philadelphia: F. A. Davis, 1975.

Dunn, A. J., and S. C. Bondy. *Functional Chemistry of the Brain*. Flushing, N. Y.: Spectrum, 1974.

Emery, A. E. H. *Elements of Medical Genetics*. 4th ed. Berkeley: University of California Press, 1975.

Fast, J. *Blueprint For Life: The Story of Modern Genetics*. New York: St. Martin's Press, 1964.

Fletcher, J. *The Ethics of Genetic Control: Ending Reproductive Roulette*. Garden City, N.Y.: Anchor Press, 1974.

Frankl, V. E. *Man's Search for Meaning: An Introduction to Logotherapy*. London: Hodder and Stoughton, 1964.

Gould Medical Dictionary. 3rd ed. New York: McGraw-Hill, 1972.

Hsia, Y. E., et al., eds. *Counseling in Genetics*. New York: Alan R. Liss, Inc., 1979.

Huntington's (Chorea) Disease: Handbook for Health Professionals. New York: Committee to Combat Huntington's Disease, 1974.

Kessler, S., ed. *Genetic Counseling: Psychological Dimensions*. New York: Academic Press, 1979.

King, R. C. *A Dictionary of Genetics*. 2nd ed. New York: Oxford, 1972.

Kübler-Ross, E. *On Death and Dying*. New York: Macmillan, 1969.

Lenz, W. *Medical Genetics*. Chicago: University of Chicago Press, 1963.

Lubs, H. A., and F. de la Cruz, eds. *Genetic Counseling: A Monograph of the National Institute of Child Health and Human Development.* New York: Raven Press, 1977.

Lynch, H. T. *Dynamic Genetic Counseling for Clinicians.* Springfield, Ill.: C. C. Thomas, 1969.

McKusick, V. A. *Human Genetics.* 2nd ed. Englewood Cliffs, N.J.: Prentice-Hall, 1969.

McKusick, V. A. *Mendelian Inheritance in Man: Catalogs of Autosomal Dominant, Autosomal Recessive, and X-Linked Phenotypes.* 4th ed. Baltimore: Johns Hopkins Press, 1971.

McKusick, V. A., and R. Claiborne. *Medical Genetics.* New York: H.P. Publishing Co., 1973.

Milunsky, A. *The Prenatal Diagnosis of Hereditary Disorders.* Springfield, Ill.: C. C. Thomas, 1973.

Milunsky, A. *Know Your Genes.* Boston: Houghton Mifflin, 1977.

Nora, J. J., and F. C. Fraser. *Medical Genetics: Principles and Practice.* Philadelphia: Lea and Febiger, 1974.

Nyhan, W. L. *The Heredity Factor: Genes, Chromosomes, and You.* New York: Grosset and Dunlap, 1976.

Propert, D. N. "Genetic markers in the blood of healthy subjects and patients with various mental disorders." Ph.D. thesis, University of Melbourne, 1977.

Reilly, P. *Genetics, Law, and Social Policy.* Cambridge, Mass.: Harvard University Press, 1977.

Report: Commission for the Control of Huntington's Disease and Its Consequences. 10 vols. Bethesda, Md.: National Institutes of Health, 1977.

Riccardi, V. M. *The Genetic Approach to Human Disease.* New York: Oxford University Press, 1977.

Russell, W. R. *Explaining the Brain.* London: Oxford University Press, 1975.

Srb, A. M., et al., eds. *Facets of Genetics: Readings from Scientific American.* San Francisco: W. H. Freeman, 1970.

Strickberger, M. W. *Genetics.* 2nd ed. New York: MacMillan, 1976.

Sturtevant, A. H. *A History of Genetics.* New York: Harper and Row, 1965.

Sutton, H. E. *An Introduction to Human Genetics.* New York: Holt, Rinehart and Winston, 1965.

Teyler, T. J. *A Primer of Psychobiology: Brain and Behavior.* San Francisco: W. H. Freeman and Co., 1975.

Thomson, W. A. R., ed. *Black's Medical Dictionary.* 31st ed. London: Adam and Charles Black, 1976.

Vinken, P. J., and G. W. Bruyn, eds. *Handbook of Clinical Neurology.*

Vol. 6. *Diseases of the Basal Ganglia.* Amsterdam: North-Holland Publishing Co., 1968.

ARTICLES

Albano, C., and L. Cocito. "Huntington's chorea and bromocriptine" (letter). *Archives of Neurology* 36.5 (May 1979):322.

Altman, L. K. "Birth-defect suits worry doctors." *New York Times*, 30 January 1979.

Aminoff, M. J., and M. Gross. "Vasoregulatory activity in patients with Huntington's chorea." *Journal of the Neurological Sciences* 21.1 (January 1974):33–38.

Aminoff, M.J., et al. "Pattern of intellectual impairment in Huntington's chorea." *Psychological Medicine* 5.2 (May 1975):169–72.

"Annual Report, 1977–1978." New York: National Huntington's Disease Association, 1978.

Aquilonius, S. M. "Research in hereditary chorea—an update." *Acta Neurologica Scandinavica* (supplement) 57.67 (1978):115–22.

Aquilonius, S. M., and R. Sjöström. "Cholinergic and dopaminergic mechanisms in Huntington's chorea." *Life Sciences* 1.10.7 (1 April 1971):405–14.

Aquilonius, S. M., et al. "Regional distribution of choline acetyltransferase in the human brain: changes in Huntington's chorea." *Journal of Neurology, Neurosurgery and Psychiatry* 38.7 (July 1975):669–77.

Attwood, A. "Dead singer's fight goes on." *The Age* (Melbourne), 2 November 1979.

Barbeau, A. "L-DOPA and juvenile Huntington's disease" (letter). *Lancet* 2.629 (15 November 1969):1066.

Barbeau, A. "Parental ascent in the juvenile form of Huntington's chorea" (letter). *Lancet* 2.679 (31 October 1970):937.

Barbeau, A. "GABA and Huntington's chorea" (letter). *Lancet* 2.844 (29 December 1973): 1499–1500.

Barbeau, A. "Progress in understanding Huntington's chorea." *Canadian Journal of Neurological Sciences* 2.2 (May 1975): 81–85.

Barbeau, A. "Recent developments in Parkinson's disease and Huntington's chorea." *International Journal of Neurology* 11.1 (1976):17–27.

Barbeau, A. "Quebec cooperative study of Friedreich's Ataxia: design of the investigation." *Canadian Journal of Neurological Sciences* 3.4 (November 1976):271–74.

Barbeau, A. "Friedreich's Ataxia 1979: an overview." *Canadian Journal of Neurological Sciences* 6.2 (May 1979):311–19.

Barbeau, A., and K. Ando. "Dopamine and Huntington's chorea" (letter). *Lancet* 1.7913 (26 April 1975):987.

Barbeau, A., et al. "La chorée de Huntingdon chez les Canadiens Français." *Union Médicale de Canada* 93 (1964):1178.

Barber, R. "Huntington's chorea." *Nursing Times* 74.28 (13 July 1978): 1165–67.

Barkley, D. S., et al. "Huntington's disease: delayed hypersensitivity in vitro to human central nervous system antigens." *Science* 195.4275 (21 January 1977):314–16.

Beckman, L., et al. "Association and linkage studies of Huntington's chorea in relation to fifteen genetic markers." *Hereditas* 77.1 (1974): 73–80.

Behan, P., and I. Bone. "Hereditary chorea without dementia." *Journal of Neurology, Neurosurgery, and Psychiatry* 40.7 (July 1977):687–91.

Bell, J. "Huntington's chorea." In *The Treasury of Human Inheritance*, vol. 4, edited by R. A. Fisher and L. S. Penrose, pp. 1–29. London: Cambridge University Press, 1948.

Bell, R. D. "Huntington's chorea." Paper delivered at the Huntington's Disease Symposium, The University of Texas Health Science Center at San Antonio, 1979.

Belson, A. "Little-known disease." *Family Health* 9 (May 1977).

Bergsma, D., ed. "Contemporary genetic counseling: proceedings of a symposium of the American Society of Human Genetics." *Birth Defects* (original article series) 9.4 (April 1973).

Bird, E. D. "Biochemical studies on gamma-aminobutyric acid metabolism in Huntington's chorea." In *Biochemistry and Neurology*, edited by H. F. Bradford and C. D. Marsden, pp. 83–92. London: Academic Press, 1976.

Bird, E. D. "The brain in Huntington's chorea." *Psychological Medicine* 8.3 (August 1978):357–60.

Bird, E. D., and L. L. Iversen. "Rigidity in Huntington's chorea" (letter). *Lancet* 1.855 (16 March 1974):463.

Bird, E. D., and L. L. Iversen. "Huntington's chorea: post-mortem measurement of glutamic acid decarboxylase, choline acetyltransferase and dopamine in basal ganglia." *Brain* 97.3 (September 1974):457–72.

Bird, E. D., et al. "Reduced glutamic-acid-decarboxylase activity in Huntington's chorea." *Lancet* 1.812 (19 May 1973):1090–92.

Bird, E. D., et al. "A sex-related factor in the inheritance of Huntington's chorea." *Annals of Human Genetics* 37.3 (January 1974):255–60.

Bird, E. D., et al. "Penicillamine in Huntington's chorea." *Postgraduate Medical Journal* (supplement) 2 (August 1974):24–26.

Bird, M. T., and G. W. Paulson. "The rigid form of Huntington's chorea." *Neurology* 21.3 (March 1971):271–76.

Bird, T. D. "Normal glutamic acid decarboxylase activity in kidney tissue from patients with Huntington's disease." *Journal of Neurochemistry* 27.6 (December 1976):155–57.

Bird, T. D., and G. S. Omenn. "Monozygotic twins with Huntington's disease in a family expressing the rigid variant." *Neurology* 25.12 (December 1975):1126–29.

Bittenbender, J. B., and F. A. Quadfasel. "Rigid and akinetic forms of Huntington's chorea." *Archives of Neurology* 7 (1962):275–78.

Bjorklund, J. H. "HD victims: all is not gloom." *San Francisco Sunday Examiner and Chronicle*, 30 October 1977.

Boll, T. J., et al. "Neuropsychological and emotional correlates of Huntington's chorea." *Journal of Nervous and Mental Disease* 158.1 (January 1974):61–69.

Bolt, J. M. W. "Abortion and Huntington's chorea" (letter). *British Medical Journal* 1.595 (30 March 1968):840.

Bolt, J. M. W. "Huntington's chorea in the west of Scotland." *British Medical Journal* 116.532 (March 1970):259–70.

Bolt, J. M. W., and G. P. Lewis. "Huntington's chorea: a study of liver function and histology." *Quarterly Journal of Medicine* 42.165 (January 1973):151–74.

Brackenridge, C. J. "A genetic and statistical study of some sex-related factors in Huntington's disease." *Clinical Genetics* 2.5 (1971):267–86.

Brackenridge, C. J. "Relation of type of initial symptoms and line of transmission to ages at onset and death in Huntington's disease." *Clinical Genetics* 2.5 (1971):287–97.

Brackenridge, C. J. "Familial correlations for age of onset and age of death in Huntington's disease." *Journal of Medical Genetics* 9.1 (March 1972):23–32.

Brackenridge, C. J. "The relation of sex of affected parent to the age at onset of Huntington's disease." *Journal of Medical Genetics* 10.4 (December 1973):333–36.

Brackenridge, C. J. "Relation of parental age to rigidity in Huntington's disease." *Journal of Medical Genetics* 11.2 (June 1974):136–40.

Brackenridge, C. J., and B. Teltscher. "Estimation of the age at onset of Huntington's disease from factors associated with the affected parent." *Journal of Medical Genetics* 12.1 (March 1975):64–69.

Brackenridge, C. J., et al. "A linkage study of the loci for Huntington's disease and some common polymorphic markers." *Annals of Human Genetics* 42.2 (October 1978):203–11.

Brothers, C. R. D. "The history and incidence of Huntington's chorea in Tasmania." *Royal Australasian College of Physicians* 4 (January 1949):48–50.

Brothers, C. R. D., and A. W. Meadows. "An investigation of Huntington's chorea in Victoria." *Journal of Mental Science* 101 (1955):548.

Bruyn, G. W. "Neuropathology of Huntington's disease." Paper delivered at the First Australian Huntington's Disease Conference, Balwyn, Victoria, 2 November 1979.

Bruyn, G. W., and W. J. A. von Wolferen. "Pathogenesis of Huntington's chorea" (letter). *Lancet* 1.816 (16 June 1973):1382.

Burke, W. "Age of onset in Huntington's disease: lack of parental age effect." *Journal of Medical Genetics* 13.6 (October 1976):462–65.

Butterfield, D. A., et al. "Electron spin resonance study of membrane protein alterations in erythrocytes in Huntington's disease." *Nature* 267.5610 (2 June 1977):453–55.

Butters, N., et al. "Comparison of the neuropsychological deficits associated with early and advanced Huntington's disease." *Archives of Neurology* 35.9 (September 1978):585–89.

Butterworth, R. F., et al. "Platelet dopamine uptake in Huntington's chorea and Gilles de la Tourette's syndrome: effect of haloperidol." *Canadian Journal of Neurological Sciences* 4.4 (November 1977):285–88.

Buxton, M. "Diagnostic problems in Huntington's chorea and tardive dyskinesia." *Comprehensive Psychiatry* 17.2 (1976):325–33.

Byers, R. K., and J. A. Dodge. "Huntington's chorea in children: report of four cases." *Neurology* 17.6 (June 1967):587–96.

Byers, R. K., et al. "Huntington's disease in children: neuropathologic study of four cases." *Neurology* 23.6 (June 1973):561–69.

Caine, E. D., et al. "An outline for the analysis of dementia: the memory disorder in Huntington's disease." *Neurology* 27.11 (November 1977):1087–92.

Caine, E. D., et al. "Huntington's dementia: clinical and neuropsychological features." *Archives of General Psychiatry* 35.3 (March 1978):377–84.

Caine, E. D., et al. "Neuroendocrine function in Huntington's disease: dopaminergic regulation of prolactin release." *Life Sciences* 22.10 (March 1978):911–18.

Caraceni, T., et al. "Study of the excitability cycle of the blink reflex in Huntington's chorea." *European Neurology* 14.6 (November 1976):465–72.

Caraceni, T., et al. "Biochemical aspects of Huntington's chorea." *Journal of Neurology, Neurosurgery and Psychiatry* 40.6 (June 1977):581–87.

Caraceni, T., et al. "Pharmacology of Huntington's chorea: personal experience." *European Neurology* 16 (December 1977):42–50.

Caro, A. "The prevalence of Huntington's chorea in an area of East Anglia." *Journal of the Royal College of General Practitioners* 27.166 (January 1977):41–45.

Caro, A., et al. "Genetic counseling in Huntington's chorea" (letter). *British Medical Journal* 2.6026 (3 July 1976):46.

Catchpole, D. "Our life with Huntington's chorea." *Nursing Times* 70.42 (17 October 1974):1616–18.

Cederbaum, S. "Tests for Huntington's chorea" (letter). *New England Journal of Medicine* 284.18 (6 May 1971):1045.

Chandler, J. H. "EEG in prediction of Huntington's chorea: an eighteen year follow-up." *Electroencephalography and Clinical Neurophysiology* 21.1 (July 1966):79–80.

Chase, T. N. "Rational approaches to the pharmacotherapy of chorea." *Research Publications of the Association for Research in Nervous and Mental Disease* 55 (1976):337–50.

Chase, T. N., et al. "Huntington's chorea: effect of serotonin depletion." *Archives of Neurology* 26.3 (March 1972):282–84.

Chiu, E. "Notes on the management of Huntington's disease." *Australian Family Physician* 8.2 (February 1979):197–99.

Chiu, E., and B. Teltscher. "Huntington's disease: the establishment of a national register." *Medical Journal of Australia* 2.8 (7 October 1978): 394–96.

Clow, C. L. "On the application of knowledge to the patient with genetic disease." In *Progress in Medical Genetics*, vol. 9, edited by A. G. Steinberg and A. G. Bearn, pp. 159–213. New York: Grune and Stratton, 1973.

Coyle, J. T., and R. Schwarez. "Lesion of striatal neurons with kainic acid provides a model for Huntington's chorea." *Nature* 263 (16 September 1976):244–46.

Coyle, J. T., et al. "Clinical neuropathologic and pharmacologic aspects of Huntington's disease: correlates with a new animal model." *Progress in Neuropsychopharmacology* 1.1–2(1977):13–20.

Crick, F. H. C. "Thinking about the brain." *Scientific American* 241.3 (September 1979):181–88.

Critchely, M. "Huntington's chorea in East Anglia." *Journal of State Medicine* 42 (1934):575.

Davis, A. "Nursing care study: Emily—a victim of Huntington's chorea." *Nursing Times* 72.12 (25 March 1976):449–50.

Davis, K. L., et al. "Choline in tardive dyskinesia and Huntington's disease." *Life Sciences* 19.10 (15 November 1976):1507–15.

"Decade of progress and hope, 1967–1977." New York: Committee to Combat Huntington's Disease, 1977.

Dewhurst, K. E. "Personality disorder in Huntington's disease." *Psychiatria Clinica* 3.4 (1970):221–29.

Dewhurst, K. E., and J. E. Oliver. "Huntington's disease of young people." *European Neurology* 3.5 (1970):278–89.

Dewhurst, K. E., et al. "Neuro-psychiatric aspects of Huntington's disease." *Confinia Neurologica* 31.4 (1969):258–68.

Dewhurst, K. E., et al. "Socio-psychiatric consequences of Huntington's disease." *British Journal of Psychiatry* 116.532 (March 1970):255–58.

"Dopamine and GABA in Huntington's chorea: editorial." *Lancet* 2.7889 (9 November 1974):1122–23.

Elliotson, J. "St. Vitus' dance." *Lancet* 1 (1832):161.

Enna, S. J., et al. "Huntington's chorea: changes in neurotransmitter receptors in the brain." *New England Journal of Medicine* 294.24 (10 June 1976):1305–9.

Enna, S. J., et al. "Alterations of brain neurotransmitter receptor binding in Huntington's chorea." *Brain Research* 116.3 (12 November 1976): 531–37.

Enna, S. J., et al. "Neurobiology and pharmacology of Huntington's disease." *Life Sciences* 20.2 (15 January 1977):205–11.

Enna, S. J., et al. "Cerebrospinal fluid gamma-aminobutyric acid variations in neurological disorders." *Archives of Neurology* 34.11 (November 1977):683–85.

Erdomez, D. "Music therapy in Huntington's disease." Paper delivered at the First Australian Huntington's Disease Conference, Balwyn, Victoria, November 1979.

Fahn, S. "L-DOPA effect in Huntington's chorea." *New England Journal of Medicine* 287.9 (31 August 1972):467–68.

Fahn, S. "Workshop report on research commission on Huntington's chorea of the World Federation of Neurology, Leiden, The Netherlands." New York: Committee to Combat Huntington's Disease, September 1977.

Fraser, F. C. "Genetic counseling." *Hospital Practice* 6.1 (January 1971):49–56.

Fraser, F. C. "Genetic counseling." *American Journal of Human Genetics* 26 (1974):636–59.

Free, J. W., and C. McPhillips. "Huntington's disease: how to solve its unique care problems." *RN* 40.8 (August 1977):44–47.

Freemon, F. R. "Pretesting for Huntington's disease: another view." *Hastings Center Report: Institute of Society Ethics and the Life Sciences* 3.4 (September 1973):13.

Gale, F., and J. H. Bennett. "Huntington's chorea in a South Australian community of aboriginal descent." *Medical Journal of Australia* 2.10 (6 September 1969):482–84.

Gale, J. S., et al. "Human brain substance P: distribution in controls and Huntington's chorea." *Journal of Neurochemistry* 30:3 (March 1978):633–34.

Galton, L. "Researchers zero in on a 'diabolical' disease." *Parade*, 17 December 1978.

"Genetic counseling: report of an ad hoc committee of the American

Society of Human Genetics." *American Journal of Human Genetics* 27.2 (March 1975):240–42.

Glaeser, B. S., et al. "GABA levels in cerebrospinal fluid of patients with Huntington's chorea: a preliminary report." *Biochemical Medicine* 12.4 (April 1975):380–85.

Goebel, H. H., et al. "Juvenile Huntington chorea: clinical, ultrastructural and biochemical studies." *Neurology* 28.1 (January 1978):23–31.

Goetz, C. G., and W. J. Weiner. "Huntington's disease: current concepts of therapy." *Journal of the American Geriatrics Society* 27.1 (January 1979):23–26.

Goetz, I., et al. "Fibroblasts in Huntington's disease." *New England Journal of Medicine* 293.24 (11 December 1975):1225–27.

Goodman, R. M., et al. "Huntington's chorea: a multidisciplinary study of affected parents and first generation offspring." *Archives of Neurology* 15.4 (October 1966):345–55.

"Guthries face a cloudy future." *Wichita Eagle and Beacon*, 6 May 1979.

Hans, M. B., and T. H. Gilmore. "Social aspects of Huntington's chorea." *British Journal of Psychiatry* 114.506 (January 1968):93–98.

Hans, M. B., and T. H. Gilmore. "Huntington's chorea and genealogical credibility." *Journal of Nervous and Mental Disease* 148.1 (January 1969):5–13.

Hansotia, P., et al. "Juvenile Huntington's chorea." *Neurology* 18.3 (March 1968):217–24.

Hayes, L., et al. "A study of the needs for care of Huntington's disease patients and their families in the Sydney metropolitan area." Sydney: unpublished report, October, 1980, pp. 1–32.

Heathfield, K. W. G. "Huntington's chorea: investigation into the prevalence of this disease in the area covered by the North East Metropolitan Regional Hospital Board." *Brain: Journal of Neurology* 90.1 (March 1967):203–32.

Heathfield, K. W. G. "Huntington's chorea: a centenary review." *Postgraduate Medical Journal* 49.567 (January 1973):32–45.

Hecht, F., and L. B. Holmes. "What we don't know about genetic counseling." *New England Journal of Medicine* 287.9 (31 August 1972):464–65.

Hemphill, M. "Pretesting for Huntington's disease: an overview." *Hastings Center Report: Institute of Society, Ethics and the Life Sciences* 3.3 (June 1973):12–13.

"Hereditary disease." Beverly Hills, California: Hereditary Disease Foundation, n.d.

Higgins, R. "Huntington's chorea." *Nursing Times* 72.30 (29 July 1976):1164–65.

Huang, C. Y., et al. "Tetrabenazine in the treatment of Huntington's chorea." *Medical Journal of Australia* 1.16 (17 April 1976):583–84.

Huntington, G. "On chorea." *The Medical and Surgical Reporter* 26.15 (13 April 1872):317–21.

"Huntington's chorea." London: Committee on Huntington's Chorea of the Central Council of the Disabled, n.d.

"Huntington's chorea." *Lancet* 2.512 (19 August 1967):409–10.

"Huntington's chorea." *Canadian Medical Association Journal* 102.10 (23 May 1970):1106.

"Huntington's chorea." *British Medical Journal* 1.717 (1 August 1970):238.

"Huntington's chorea." *Lancet* 1.8013 (26 March 1977):702–3.

"Huntington's disease: an animal model." *Science News* 110 (October 1976).

"Huntington's disease (Huntington's chorea)." Bethesda, Md: United States Department of Health, Education, and Welfare, National Institutes of Health, 1976.

Iqbal, K., et al. "Protein abnormalities in Huntington's chorea." *Brain Research* 76.1 (9 August 1974):178–84.

Iverson, L. L. "The chemistry of the brain." *Scientific American* 241.3 (September 1979):118–29.

Iverson, L. L., et al. "Analysis of glutamate decarboxylase in post-mortem brain tissue in Huntington's chorea." *Journal of Psychiatric Research* 11 (1974):255–56.

James, W. E., et al. "Early signs of Huntington's chorea." *Diseases of the Nervous System* 30.8 (August 1969):556–59.

Jervis, G. A. "Huntington's chorea in childhood." *Archives of Neurology* 9 (1963):244–57.

Johnson, K. E. "Nursing care study. Huntington's chorea: a one in two chance of dying." *Nursing Mirror* 147.21 (23 November 1978):20–31.

Johnston, G. A. R. "Glutamic acid and Huntington's disease." Paper delivered at the First Australian Huntington's Disease Conference, Balwyn, Victoria, 2 November 1979.

Kelly, J. "Nursing care study. Huntington's chorea: a mother shunned by her family." *Nursing Mirror* 148.15 (12 April 1979):45–46.

Keogh, H. J., et al. "Altered growth hormone release in Huntington's chorea." *Journal of Neurology, Neurosurgery and Psychiatry* 39:3 (March 1976):244–48.

Kirk, D., et al. "Anomalous cellular proliferation in vitro associated with Huntington's disease." *Human Genetics* 36.2 (15 April 1977):143–54.

Klawans, H. L. "Toward an understanding of the pathophysiology of

Huntington's chorea." *Confinia Neurologica* 33.5 (1971):297–303.

Klawans, H. L., and M. M. Cohen. "Diseases of the extrapyramidal system." *Disease-a-Month* (January 1970):44–52.

Klawans, H. L., et al. "Predictive test for Huntington's chorea" (letter). *Lancet* 2.684 (5 December 1970):1185–86.

Klawans, H. L., et al. "Use of L-DOPA in the detection of presymptomatic Huntington's chorea." *New England Journal of Medicine* 286.25 (June 1972):1332–34.

Klawans, H. L., et al. "Recent advances in the biochemical pharmacology of extrapyramidal movement disorders." *Advances in Experimental Medicine and Biology* 90 (1977):21–47.

Klawans, H. L., et al. "Levodopa and presymptomatic detection of Huntington's disease—eight-year follow-up." *New England Journal of Medicine* 302:19 (8 May 1980):1090.

Korenyi, C., and J. R. Whittier. "Huntington's disease (chorea) in New York state: approximate gene prevalence in New York City and on Long Island." *New York State Journal of Medicine* 77.1 (January 1977):44–45.

Korenyi, C., et al. "Stress in Huntington's disease (chorea): review of the literature and personal observations." *Diseases of the Nervous System* 33.5 (May 1972):339–44.

Lane, C. S. "Walk a dark vale: Huntington's chorea." *Nursing Care* 9.5 (May 1976):30–31.

Leonard, C. O., et al. "Genetic counseling: a consumers' view." *New England Journal of Medicine* 287.9 (31 August 1972):433–39.

Linnen, B. "Marjorie Guthrie sings out against cause of Woody's death." *Minnesota Daily*, 14 October 1977.

Little, L. "Guthrie family one of many stalked by disease." *The Dallas Morning News*, 15 August 1976.

Lloyd, K. G., et al. "Alterations in 3H-GABA binding in Huntington's chorea." *Life Sciences* 21.5 (1 September 1977):747–53.

Llye, O., and I. I. Gottesman. "Premorbid psychometric indicators of the gene for Huntington's disease." *Journal of Consulting and Clinical Psychology* 45.6 (December 1977):1011–22.

Llye, O., and W. Quast. "The bender gestalt: use of clinical judgment versus recall scores in prediction in Huntington's disease." *Journal of Consulting and Clinical Psychology* 44.2 (April 1976):229–32.

Loeb, C., et al. "Levodopa and Huntington's chorea." *Journal of Neurology, Neurosurgery and Psychiatry* 39.10 (October 1976):958–61.

Lynch, H. T., et al. "Subjective perspective of a family with Huntington's disease: implications for genetic counseling." *Archives of General Psychiatry* 27.1 (July 1972):67–72.

Lyon, R. LL. "Huntington's chorea in the Moray Firth area." *British Medical Journal* 5288 (12 May 1962):1301–6.

McGeer, E. G., and P. L. McGeer. "Duplication of biochemical changes of Huntington's chorea by intrastriatal injections of glutamic and kainic acids." *Nature* 263 (7 October 1976):517–18.

McGeer, P. L., and E. G. McGeer. "Enzymes associated with the metabolism of catecholamines, acetylcholine and GABA in human controls and patients with Parkinson's disease and Huntington's chorea." *Journal of Neurochemistry* 26.1 (January 1976):65–76.

McGeer, P. L., and E. G. McGeer. "The GABA system and function of the basal ganglia: Huntington's disease." In *GABA in Nervous System Function*, edited by E. Roberts, et al. New York: Raven Press, 1976.

McGeer, P. L., et al. "Choline acetylase and glutamic acid decarboxylase in Huntington's chorea: a preliminary study." *Neurology* 23.9 (September 1973):912–17.

MacKay, C. R., and J. M. Shea. "Ethical considerations in research on Huntington's disease." *Clinical Research* 25.4 (October 1977):241–47.

McKusick, V. A. "Editorial: family-oriented follow-up." *Journal of Chronic Diseases* 22.1 (June 1969):1–7.

Maddison, D., and B. Raphael. "Social and psychological consequences of chronic disease in childhood." *Medical Journal of Australia* 2.3 (18 December 1971):1265–70.

Manning, M. "Combating the agony of Huntington's chorea." *Nursing Mirror* 146.9 (2 March 1978):7–9.

Markesbery, W. R., and D. A. Butterfield. "Scanning electron microscopy studies of erythrocytes in Huntington's disease." *Biochemical and Biophysical Research Communications* 78.2 (23 September 1977):560–64.

Mead, A. "Widow seeking freedom from sufferers of disease." *Fort Worth Star-Telegram*, 19 January 1979.

Menkes, J. H., and N. Stein. "Fibroblast cultures in Huntington's disease" (letter). *New England Journal of Medicine* 288.16 (19 April 1973):856–57.

Menkes, J. H., et al. "Huntington's disease: growth and fatty acid metabolism of fibroblast cultures in lipid-deficient medium." *Transactions of the American Neurological Association* 101 (1976):64–68.

Miller, E. "The social work component in community-based action on behalf of victims of Huntington's disease." *Social Work in Health Care* 2.1 (Fall 1976):25–32.

Moshell, A. N., et al. "Radiosensitivity in Huntington's disease: implications for pathogenesis and presymptomatic diagnosis." *Lancet* 1 (5 January 1980):9–11.

Myrianthopoulos, N. C. "Huntington's chorea: review article." *Journal of Medical Genetics* 3 (December 1966):298–314.

Nee, L. E., and a patient. "Experiences of a Huntington's disease patient." *Nursing Care* (May 1976).

Oliver, J. E. "Abortion and Huntington's chorea" (letter). *British Medical Journal* 1.591 (2 March 1968):576–77.

Oliver, J. E. "Huntington's chorea in Northamptonshire." *British Journal of Psychiatry* 116.532 (March 1970):241–53.

Oliver, J. E., and K. E. Dewhurst. "Childhood and adolescent forms of Huntington's disease." *Journal of Neurology, Neurosurgery and Psychiatry* 32.5 (October 1969):455–59.

Oliver, J. E., and K. E. Dewhurst. "Six generations of ill-used children in a Huntington's pedigree." *Postgraduate Medical Journal* 45.530 (December 1969):757–60.

Olney, J. W., and T. de Gubareff. "Glutamate neurotocity and Huntington's chorea." *Nature* 271 (9 February 1978):557–59.

Palmer, I. O. "Huntington's chorea." *Nursing Times* 69.32 (9 August 1973):1015–20.

Parker, N. "Observations on Huntington's chorea based on a Queensland survey." *Medical Journal of Australia* 1 (1958):351.

Patterson, R. M., et al. "The prediction of Huntington's chorea: an electroencephalographic and genetic study." *American Journal of Psychiatry* 104 (June 1948):786–97.

Paulson, G. W. "Predictive tests in Huntington's disease." *Research Publications of the Association for Research in Nervous and Mental Disease* 55 (1976):317–29.

Paulson, G. W. "A neurologist speaks with Huntington's disease families." New York: National Huntington's Disease Association, n.d.

Pearson, J. S. "Family support and counseling in Huntington's disease." *The Psychiatric Forum* (Fall 1973):46–50.

Perry, T. L. "Isoniazid and Huntington's chorea" (letter). *New England Journal of Medicine* 298.19 (11 May 1978):1092–93.

Perry, T. L., et al. "Plasma-aminoacid levels in Huntington's chorea." *Lancet* 1.599 (19 April 1969):806–8.

Perry, T. L., et al. "Huntington's chorea: deficiency of gamma-aminobutyric acid in brain." *New England Journal of Medicine* 288.7 (15 February 1973):337–42.

Perry, T. L., et al. "GABA in Huntington's chorea" (letter). *Lancet* 1.864 (18 May 1974):995–96.

Phillips, D. H. "Genetic counseling for Huntington's disease: a consumer analysis." *Australian Family Physician* 9.8 (August 1980):585–88.

Phillipson, O. T., and E. D. Bird. "Plasma growth hormone concentrations in Huntington's chorea." *Clinical Science and Molecular Medicine* 50.6 (June 1976):551–54.

Phillipson, O. T., and E. D. Bird. "Plasma glucose, non-esterified fatty acids and amino acids in Huntington's chorea." *Clinical Science and Molecular Medicine* 52.3 (March 1977):311–18.

Pinel, C. "Huntington's chorea." *Nursing Times* 72.12 (25 March 1976): 447–48.

Podolsky, S., and N. A. Leopold. "Abnormal glucose tolerance and arginine tolerance tests in Huntington's disease." *Gerontology* 23.1 (1977):55–63.

Powledge, T. M., and J. Fletcher. "Guidelines for the ethical, social and legal issues in prenatal diagnosis." *New England Journal of Medicine* 300 (25 January 1979):168–72.

"Predictive tests in Huntington's chorea" (editorial). *British Medical Journal* 1.6112 (4 March 1978):528–29.

"Presymptomatic detection of Huntington's chorea." *British Medical Journal* 3.826 (2 September 1972):540.

Propert, D. N. "Presymptomatic detection of Huntington's disease." *Medical Journal of Australia* 1 (14 June 1980):609–12.

Reed, S. C. "A short history of genetic counseling." *Social Biology* 21.4 (Winter 1974):332–39.

Reisine, T. D., et al. "Alterations in dopaminergic receptors in Huntington's disease." *Life Sciences* 21.8 (15 October 1977):1123–28.

Roberts, E., et al. "A note on experimental approaches to Huntington's disease." *Research Publications of the Association for Research in Nervous and Mental Disease* 55 (1976):331–36.

Rosenberg, S., et al. "Detection of presymptomatic carriers of Huntington's chorea." *Neuropsychobiology* 3 (1977):144–52.

Rothstein, E. "Huntington's chorea: optimistic view" (letter). *New England Journal of Medicine* 285.13 (23 September 1971):751.

Schwarcz, R., et al. "Loss of striatal serotonin synaptic receptor binding induced by kainic acid lesions: correlations with Huntington's disease." *Journal of Neurochemistry* 28.4 (April 1977):867–69.

Scott, D. F., et al. "The EEG in Huntington's chorea: a clinical and neuropathological study." *Journal of Neurology, Neurosurgery and Psychiatry* 35.1 (February 1972):97–102.

"Secrets of the human cell." *Newsweek* 94.8 (international ed., 20 August 1979):42–48.

Segal, M. "Predictive tests in Huntington's chorea" (letter). *British Medical Journal* 1.6116 (1 April 1978):859.

Shaffer, R. A. "Mastering the mind." *Wall Street Journal*, 12 August 1977.

Shokeir, M. H. "Investigations on Huntington's disease in the Canadian prairies." *Clinical Genetics* 7.4 (April 1975):345–60.

Shoulson, I., and T. N. Chase. "Huntington's disease." *Annual Review of Medicine* 26 (1975):419–26.

Shoulson, I., and S. Fahn. "Huntington's disease: clinical care and evaluation." *Neurology* 29.1 (January 1979):1–3.

Shoulson, I., et al. "Huntington's disease: treatment with imidazole-4-acetic acid." *New England Journal of Medicine* 293.10 (4 September 1975):504–5.

Shoulson, I., et al. "Clinical care of the patient and family with Huntington's disease." (New York: Committee to Combat Huntington's Disease, 1978).

Sishta, S. K., et al. "Huntington's chorea: an electroencephalographic and psychometric study." *Electroencephalography and Clinical Neurophysiology* 36.4 (April 1974):387–93.

Smith, A. "Fear at prospect of disabling disease drives wedge into lives of families." *Birmingham News*, 17 December 1978.

Smith, C., et al. "Individuals at risk in families with genetic disease." *Journal of Medical Genetics* 8.4 (December 1971):453–59.

Spokes, E. G. S. "Neurochemical alterations in Huntington's chorea: a study of post-mortem brain tissue." *Brain* 103 (1980):179–210.

Stahl, W. L., and P. D. Swanson. "Biochemical abnormalities in Huntington's chorea brains." *Neurology* 24.9 (September 1974):813–19.

Stern, R., and R. Eldridge. "Attitudes of patients and their relatives to Huntington's disease." *Journal of Medical Genetics* 12.3 (September 1975):217–23.

Stevens, C. F. "The neuron." *Scientific American* 241.3 (September 1979):49–59.

Stevens, D. L. "Tests for Huntington's chorea" (letter). *New England Journal of Medicine* 285.7 (12 August 1971):413–14.

Stevens, D. L. "The history of Huntington's chorea." *Journal of the Royal College of Physicians of London* 6.3 (April 1972):271–82.

Teltscher, B., and B. Davies. "Medical and social problems of Huntington's disease." *Medical Journal of Australia* 1.7 (12 February 1972): 307–10.

Teltscher, B., and S. Polgar. "Predictive test and Huntington's disease: attitudes of 'at risk' persons to such a test." Paper delivered at the First Australian Huntington's Disease Conference, Balwyn, Victoria, 2–5 November 1979.

Terrence, C. F., et al. "Computed tomography for Huntington's disease." *Neuroradiology* 13.4 (27 June 1977):173–75.

Tolliss, W. "Nursing care study: Huntington's chorea." *Nursing Mirror* 142.22 (27 May 1976):54–55.

Tourian, A. Y., and Wu-Yen Hung. "Membrane abnormalities of Huntington's chorea fibroblasts in culture." *Biochemical and Biophysical Research Communications* 78.4 (24 October 1977):1296–1303.

Urquhart, N., et al. "GABA content and glutamic acid decarboxylase activity in brain of Huntington's chorea patients and control subjects." *Journal of Neurochemistry* 24.5 (May 1975):1071–75.

Vann, D. "Successful hypnotherapy for anxiety neurosis in Huntington's chorea." *Medical Journal of Australia* 2.3 (17 July 1971):166.

Vegter-Van Der Vlis, M., et al. "Ages of death of children with Huntington's chorea and of their affected parents." *Annals of Human Genetics* 39.3 (January 1976):329–34.

Vessie, P. R. "On the transmission of Huntington's chorea for 300 years: the Bures family group." *Journal of Nervous and Mental Disorders* 76 (1932):553–73.

Wallace, D. C. "Huntington's chorea: a partial model of the ageing process." *Medical Journal of Australia* 2.25 (18 December 1971):1275–76.

Wallace, D. C. "Huntington's chorea in Queensland: a not uncommon disease." *Medical Journal of Australia* 1.7 (12 February 1972):299–307.

Wallace, D. C. "The social effect of Huntington's chorea on reproductive effectiveness." *Annals of Human Genetics* 39.3 (January 1976):375–79.

Wallace, D. C. "Workshop on Huntington's chorea, Tel Aviv, April 1976." *Medical Journal of Australia* 1 (1977):458–59.

Wallace, D. C., and A. C. Hall. "Evidence of genetic heterogeneity in Huntington's chorea." *Journal of Neurology, Neurosurgery and Psychiatry* 35.6 (December 1972):789–800.

Walls, R. S., and P. Godfrey. "Hypersensitivity of brain tissue in Huntington's disease." Paper delivered at the First Australian Huntington's Disease Conference, Balwyn, Victoria, November 1979.

Walters, L. "Human in vitro fertilization: a review of the ethical literature." *Hastings Center Report: Institute of Society, Ethics and the Life Sciences* 9.4 (August 1974):23–43.

Wastek, G. J., et al. "Huntington's disease: regional alteration in muscarinic cholinergic receptor binding in human brain." *Life Sciences* 19.7 (1 October 1976):1033–39.

Wells, R. W. "Huntington's chorea: seeing beyond the disease." *American Journal of Nursing* 72 (1972):954–56.

Wexler, N. S. "Genetic 'Russian roulette': the experience of being 'at risk' for Huntington's disease." In *Genetic Counseling: Psychological Dimensions*, edited by S. Kessler. New York: Academic Press, 1979, pp. 397–420.

Whittier, J. R. "Treatment of Huntington's disease." *Modern Treatment* 5.2 (March 1968):332–50.

Whittier, J. R. "Prevalence of Huntington's chorea" (letter). *Journal of the American Medical Association* 226.12 (17 December 1973):1465–66.

Whittier, J. R., et al. "Effect of imipramine (tofrānil) on depression and hyperkinesia in Huntington's disease." *American Journal of Psychiatry* 118.1 (July 1961):79.

Whittier, J. R., et al. "The psychiatrist and Huntington's disease (chorea)." *American Journal of Psychiatry* 128.12 (17 June 1972):1546–50.

Index

DESIGNED BY IRVING PERKINS ASSOCIATES
COMPOSED BY FIVE STAR PHOTO TYPESETTING, INC.,
NEENAH, WISCONSIN
MANUFACTURED BY BANTA COMPANY, MENASHA, WISCONSIN
TEXT IS SET IN TIMES ROMAN
DISPLAY LINES IN STYMIE AND TIMES ROMAN

Library of Congress Cataloging in Publication Data
Phillips, Dennis H., 1940–
Living with Huntington's disease.
Bibliography: pp. 207–224
Includes index.
1. Huntington's chorea. I. Title.
RC394.H85P47   362.1'6851   81–16492
ISBN 0–299–08670–4   AACR2
ISBN 0–299–08674–7 (pbk.)